PARKSTONE LIBRARY
Britannia Road, Parkstone
Poole BH14 8AZ
Tel: 01202 742218
Email: parkstonelibrary@poole.gov.uk

1 3 APR 2019

FOR SALE

WITHDRAWN FROM STOCK

KT-431-214

Please return this item to any Poole library
by due date.

Renew on (01202) 265200 or at
www.boroughofpoole.com/libraries

boroughofpoole.com
1poolelib0814

Borough of Poole Libraries

551334083 W

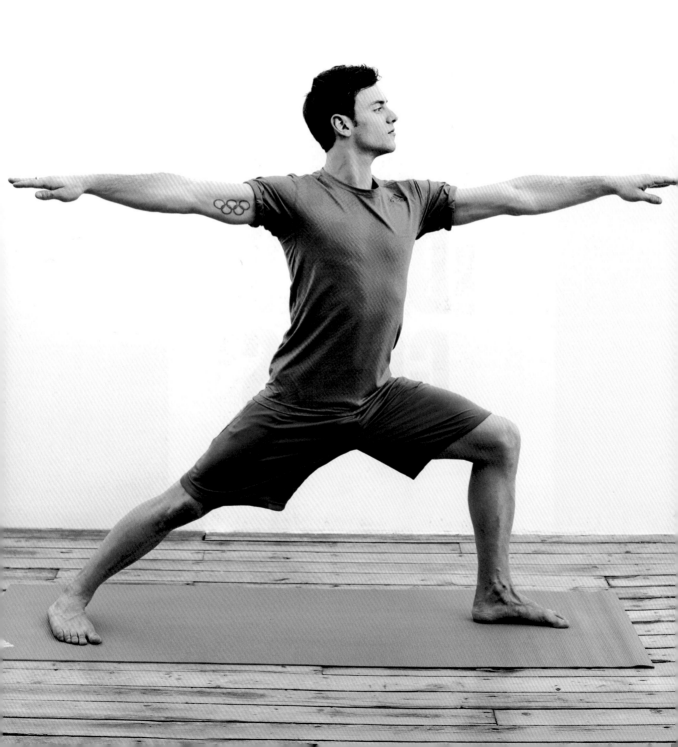

I dedicate this book to my loving husband and future family,
for their unconditional love and support

Never feel hungry
or tired again

TOM'S
DAILY
GOALS

7 easy steps to live your best life

TOM DALEY

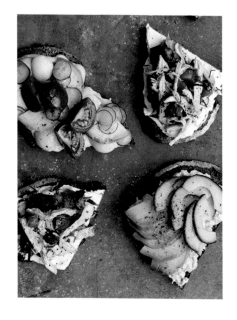
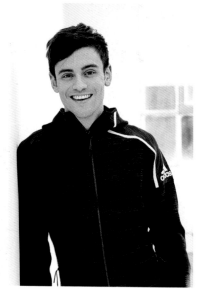
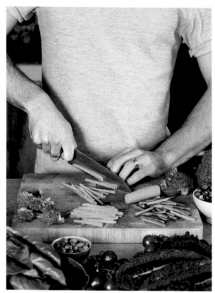

CONTENTS

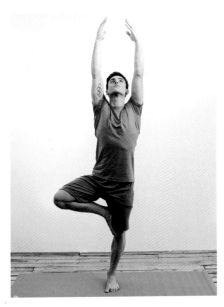
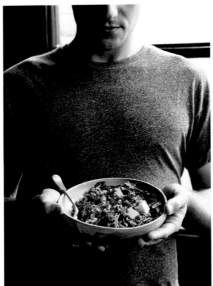
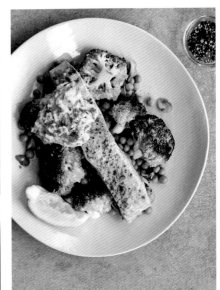

Introduction

Would you like to lead a healthier life, in which you never feel hungry or tired? One in which you can manage stress and are more resilient, productive and focused? Sometimes our goals seem so big it is hard to know where to start! Part of living a good lifestyle is transforming your knowledge or inspiration into daily habits.

This famous quote by Aristotle is a good reminder that we are the sum of our habits: 'We are what we repeatedly do. Excellence then, is not an act, but a habit.' In order to kick-start a healthier lifestyle – one in which you eat, sleep and exercise well and practise good physical and mental self-care – it is not about simply adopting a fad diet for a few weeks or promising yourself a lie-in every weekend for a month, it is about much more than this. Sometimes we start out with great intentions to get fit/lose weight/get more sleep, but all too often our attention and energy wane, we get distracted or we don't see results quickly, so we give up.

To be the best you can be, you have to treat your body and brain in the right way. As an Olympic athlete, I've not always had an easy journey but habit-forming has been key to my success. I have to take my habits and routine seriously, even though there are times when I find it very hard! From consistently getting between eight and nine hours' quality sleep a night and focusing on getting all the correct nutrients in my diet, through to prioritising meditation sessions and creating new goals and challenges, my happiness, well-being and sporting achievements are all about the small details and patterns of my life, as well as the bigger ones.

More than 40 per cent of our actions every day are not decisions but habits. The fact that habits are so integral to our daily lives means that we spend much of our day performing them. Habits are our brains' way of increasing efficiency. When we first engage in a new behaviour, our brains work hard to process new information. As we understand how a behaviour or action works, it becomes automatic and our mental energy decreases. This frees up our brainpower to take on some more important challenges.

You can take back control of your life by simply adopting new habits. In *Tom's Daily Goals*, I have detailed the seven daily habits that I value and nurture myself, and that can easily be incorporated into your day. Time is one of the best ways to trigger new habits, which is why each of my habits is associated with a certain time of day. This will help you to stick to your new routine on a daily basis. These new habits begin with doing ten minutes of yoga and stretching first thing in the morning to energise and awaken the body, through to setting your own bedtime ritual that starts an hour before your intended bedtime, helping you to relax and unwind in order to get a good night's sleep. As you start to see the rewards, be it a sense of accomplishment after exercise or a feeling of calm at the end of the day, your brain will start to anticipate these and your habits will become more engrained into your life, until they become second nature. Creating a foundation of good habits will benefit your life from today onwards. This isn't a temporary fix – it's a new and far more rewarding way of living that will yield great results. Good luck!

Tom Daley

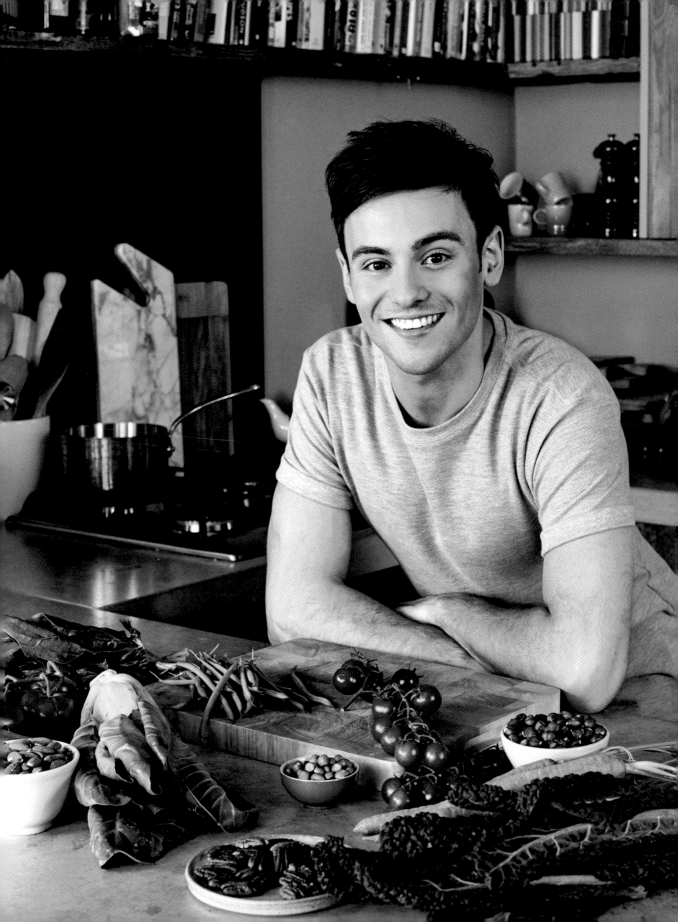

6.00

7.00

8.00

9.00

10.00

11.00

12.00

13.00

14.00

15.00

16.00

17.00

18.00

19.00

20.00

21.00

22.00

23.00

◄ **6.30** A.M.

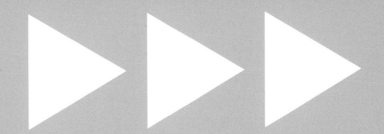

HABIT 1

MOVEMENT

What is the first thing you do when you wake up? Do you reach for your phone with bleary eyes, stagger to the shower or press the snooze button? One of the best ways to get blood flowing to the whole of your body (including your brain), improve your posture and get your metabolism moving is by practising some yoga, or simply by doing some stretches. I think what we do immediately after we wake up sets the tone for the rest of the day, so it makes sense to make this time positive, balanced and inspiring.

Yoga is an ancient form of exercise that focuses on strength, flexibility and breathing to create a unity between mind and body. Many exercise fads come and go but yoga is one that has stood the test of time; it has been around for more than 5,000 years!

There are more than 100 different types of yoga with different emphases; some are more fast-paced and intense, while others focus more on breathing and relaxation, and the intensity of your workout depends on what form you choose. The benefits of yoga are huge and well documented and there is compelling scientific proof that relaxing the mind can heal the body. It is used to increase flexibility and strength, boost immunity, prevent injury, improve balance and posture, build muscle strength, reduce stress and anxiety and improve our mind/body connection.

I first started doing Vinyasa yoga after the 2016 Olympics. When I rocked up at the first class I wasn't sure what to expect; I thought yoga would be a lazy man's workout with no real benefit but that's not the case; yoga really is for everyone of all ages and fitness abilities and can really push you. Vinyasa, which is sometimes referred to as 'breath-synchronised movement', focuses on flow and is a style of yoga that is characterised by stringing one pose to another seamlessly, using breath. You perform it at your own pace, moving in and out of postures on each inhalation or exhalation. Being aware of my breathing while I exercise has made me much more conscious of my body and of being present in the moment. I now feel and understand my body better than ever before.

Practising yoga has also really helped with my flexibility and given me more functional movement. This means training your muscles to perform everyday movements more effectively and safely, so you don't end up with a bad back, for example. By using various muscles throughout the body at the same time, it also emphasises core stability and balance, which allows me to train better. All of these benefits become more important as we get older because our muscles become tighter and shorter as we age; by practising yoga, I hope to stay strong and supple for longer. I want to be the grey-haired pensioner on the diving board!

Whether you practise some moves that you know well, or you follow a book or online routine, ten minutes of yoga poses will set you up for the day. If doing yoga doesn't appeal, just stretching out your muscles will ensure you get the blood flowing, relieve tension and calm your mind. If you sit at a computer all day, it is easy to develop bad posture as a result of poor thoracic and lumbar (upper- and lower-back) control and tight pecs (chest muscles). By stretching in the morning and taking regular breaks throughout the day you will improve alignment in your back, correct your posture and increase your flexibility.

I have included three workouts (see pages 20–43) that incorporate a mixture of Pilates and yoga exercises, including one workout for when you first get up in the morning. The wide-ranging benefits of these types of workouts are huge. They will improve your balance, posture, flexibility and range of motion and will strengthen and tone both major muscle groups and smaller ones. What's more, the mental focus and controlled breathing help to reduce stress and will improve sleep and regulate your mood. These exercises complement all the habits in this book, from helping you to become more mindful and focused, through to boosting your immunity and aiding restful and deep sleep.

My advice is to keep a yoga mat under your bed, so you can just step out of bed, pull it out and start stretching. I guarantee that ten minutes later, you will feel ready to face the day!

IF YOU DO ONE THING ...

Incorporate 10 minutes of yoga or stretching into your morning routine to awaken, energise and refresh your body and offset the effects of sitting in an office chair all day.

6 rules to get you into shape

1

Focus on all-body exercise: Yoga is great because it exercises the whole body, but by including full-body exercises, including moves like burpees, squats and press-ups during your more intense HIIT workouts, you train every major muscle group in your body. Also make sure you switch up your exercise, so if you go to the gym, make a point of using the running machine one day, the cross-trainer the next and then the rowing machine, rather than sticking to one exercise machine. You need to challenge your muscles to see results.

2

Stop making excuses: From not having the right equipment, to not having enough time, there will always be an excuse not to train. Once you get started you'll be amazed at how easy it is to form a new exercise habit. If you try to change your mindset, so exercise is not just about going to the gym and can be incorporated into your day – it can be going out for a brisk walk, playing football with friends or cycling to work – this can help.

3

Learn to be present: You must find exercise that you enjoy and discover what it means to be present. For example, when you practise yoga, concentrate on the feelings in your body and your breathing. Really breathe into the muscle or the posture you are working on and feel what is going on inside your body. Don't think about it but let your mind actually be in that body part or muscle.

We've all been guilty of starting a new exercise regime and becoming frustrated when we don't see instant results. As well as eating and exercising well, here are a few habits to help you kick-start any new fitness regime.

4

Set goals: Whether you want to learn a tricky yoga pose, or do 100 press-ups in a row, setting achievable goals will help motivate and inspire you. Ensure they are SMART (specific, measurable, achievable, relevant and timely). Write them down and plot your progress.

5

Make sure you have a rest day: Some people think that in order to get into shape you should work out seven days a week. If you are working out properly, then you need to have at least one rest day, if not two. These periods are more important than the training because they let your body repair and recover, prevent injury and allow you to keep moving forward.

6

Don't get hung up on fitness trackers: Wearable technology is becoming increasingly popular and I think it has its place because it can be a great way to figure out your limits and track progress, whether weekly, monthly or even yearly. However, I think the best way to get results is to listen to your body and pay attention to what it needs. Daily tracking of weight, progress and strength can quickly become demotivating and stressful.

Top reasons why yoga is healing

The health benefits of yoga are vast and studies continue to show that there are consistent rewards in almost every area of our health and well-being. Here are just a few ways in which it can be healing.

Boosts immunity

Yoga is one of the most effective and time-tested natural immunity boosters. It can help to stimulate the four main physiological systems that are linked to the immune system: the digestive, circulatory, endocrine and nervous systems. Poses that affect at least one of these four systems can help bolster immune function.

Increases blood flow

Like other forms of exercise, yoga gets the blood flowing around your body, improving circulation by transporting more oxygen to your cells, so they function better.

Relaxes your nervous system

Yoga makes you concentrate on the here and now, relaxing both the mind and body. It shifts the balance from the sympathetic nervous system, otherwise known as the fight-or-flight response, to the parasympathetic nervous system. This part of the nervous system slows our heart and breathing rates and is both restorative and calming.

Helps you sleep deeper

Studies suggest that regular yoga practice leads to better sleep and can help with insomnia. Yoga breathing techniques can also help you to relax and switch off.

IF YOU SUFFER FROM MIGRAINES, BACKACHE, ARTHRITIS OR OTHER CHRONIC PAIN CONDITIONS, COUNTLESS STUDIES HAVE SHOWN THAT YOGA CAN BE VERY EFFECTIVE AT REDUCING PAIN

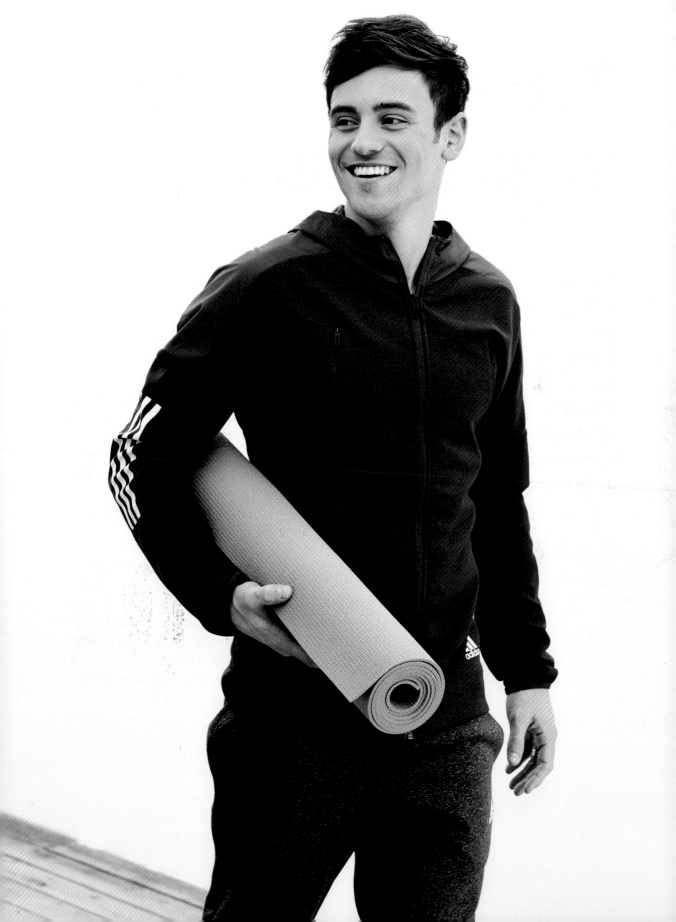

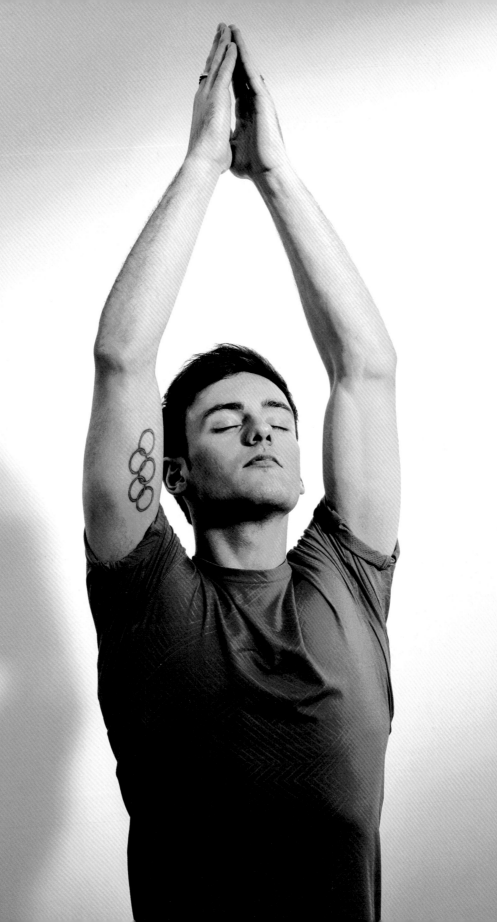

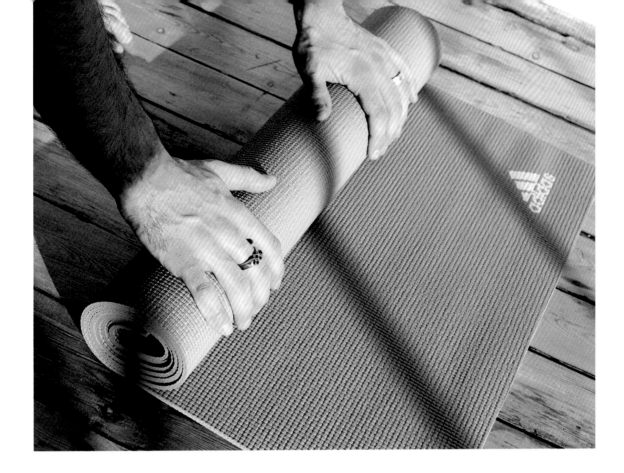

Encourages self-care

Rather than being a passive recipient of care (in the case of conventional medicine), yoga provides you with the tools to make a difference. This gives you the power to effect change; seeing improvements in your health and tuning into the positive changes in your body creates hope and optimism.

Improves self-esteem

Could your self-confidence do with a boost? Practising yoga allows the mind to relax and refocus, so you are less likely to engage in impulsive and unproductive behaviours. One Australian study showed that after a 12-week yoga programme, women who struggled with binge-eating reported improved body image and higher self-esteem.

Releases tension

Do you notice your shoulders hunched over your computer or desk? Or your hands tight around the steering wheel as you drive to work? Unconscious habits can lead to muscle fatigue and chronic tension. Doing yoga can lead to a greater awareness of your body so you will learn how to release this tension.

Workouts to boost your brain

Challenge your memory

If you're anything like me, you probably rely on your smartphone for most things. Training your memory is really easy and can be done on your daily commute: learn all the lyrics to a song in the car, or memorise the words to a poem on the Tube. Or make yourself do a task from memory, like brushing your teeth with your non-dominant hand or getting dressed in the dark.

Get lingo-happy

Language activities encourage our brains to understand, recognise and remember words. By practising language fluency your brain will be stimulated to remember old words and understand and recognise new words in context. A simple way to do this is to read outside your normal realm; rather than reading the sports section of a newspaper, read the business section, so you are exposed to new words. Learning a second language has also been proven to prevent dementia in later life.

Take a cooking class or learn to cook from scratch

Giving your brain a new experience that combines all the physical senses – taste, touch, smell, vision and hearing – can stimulate more connections between the brain areas, dramatically improving memory and making parts of the brain more resistant to ageing. A cooking class or cooking a meal from scratch is an ideal way to do this. Other examples of activities that stimulate all five senses include camping and gardening. Lance and I love to challenge each other with strange and new things all the time. Taking yourself out of your comfort zone can really awaken your senses!

Our brains are capable of some pretty amazing things and are constantly changing in response to our habits and lifestyle. It's not just our body that loses muscle over time, our brains can weaken, too. A healthy diet and regular exercise are important for brain health. In the same way that working out our bodies and using weights helps us to add lean muscle and retain muscle as we age, regular brain exercises can help increase our brain's cognitive reserve. Experts call it 'neurobic exercises' – cross-training for the brain!

Make time for friends

When you think of ways to boost your brain, hanging out with your friends probably isn't the first thing that comes to mind. However, spending time with friends and making new ones will expose you to more facts, information and ideas. Experts say that this develops our ability to focus, learn and analyse details. Practise actively listening to what other people say to expose yourself to as much new information as possible (talking to someone new on Instagram doesn't count!).

Get creative

Craft hobbies and playing board games focus the brain in the same way as meditation does. One recent study at Otago University in New Zealand showed that 'purposeful' activities, like performing music, doing arts and crafts or cooking new recipes leads to an 'upward spiral' of improved health and creativity. For example, everyone has photos on their mobile phone but what about a good old-style scrapbook? Every year I make a scrapbook of everything that has happened that year for Lance as a Christmas present. I keep tickets, passes and add photos and get creative.

THE BRAIN USES MORE ENERGY THAN ANY OTHER HUMAN ORGAN, ACCOUNTING FOR 20 PER CENT OF OUR DAILY CALORIE INTAKE

3 workouts to energise & revitalise the body & mind

These workouts are a mixture of yoga and Pilates movements and stretches that are designed to provide you with the perfect way to sync your body and mind, while at the same time giving you a workout to tone you up, using muscles you never knew you had!

We are going to target all the key muscle groups and energise and re-awaken them, so you use all of your muscles properly. I have designed these workouts to be done on alternate days, interspersed with more high-intensity cardio training of your choice, such as HIIT (high-intensity interval training), running, spinning or your normal gym training sessions, alongside one rest day. If you prefer to train very hard or are working towards a specific event, these exercises are a great way to start a session because they will activate all the smaller muscles you will need to work out most effectively.

None of these exercises requires any special equipment (all you need is a mat or a towel) and can be done in the comfort of your bedroom, living room or garden. Familiarise yourself thoroughly with all the exercises first and ensure you use the correct form and keep your core muscles engaged throughout. The key with all of these workouts is to go at your own pace, flowing through each movement with your own breathing rate. So you complete one movement on the inhalation and another on the exhalation. This can take some time to perfect and when you start off you may prefer to hold the poses for longer. Concentrating on your breath allows you to focus on the present and slowing down your breathing releases tension and stress and has a soothing effect on your emotional state.

If you are cold before working out, spend a couple of minutes shaking out your arms and legs but if you are already warm, you should be fine to start working out straight away. I make a point of never over-stretching sore areas but holding a stretch and breathing deeply until the pain eases.

THE BASICS

Here is an overview of the basic moves so you can familiarise yourself with them before you start working out properly. They will bring your mind and body together and improve both muscular and postural strength.

▶ Downward-facing Dog

One of yoga's most recognised poses, this is where the body assumes an inverted 'V' shape. Start on your hands and knees. Spread your fingers wide to distribute your weight evenly across your hands and then lift your pelvis up towards the ceiling. Keep your back straight and straighten your legs if you can, but do not lock your knees. You should feel a stretch in your hamstrings but these exercises and poses should never be painful. Relax your head and neck and try and open up your thoracic spine (the upper middle area of your back) by feeling like you are rotating your hands on the ground out from each other; you should feel some space open up.

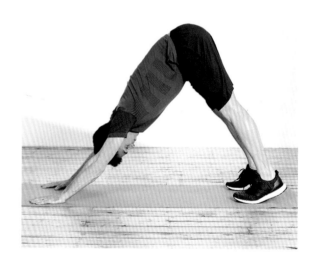

▶ Downward-facing Dog Knee Tucks

In an inverted position, lift one leg as high as you can behind you and then tuck it as far under the chest as you can. Return the leg back and repeat with the other leg.

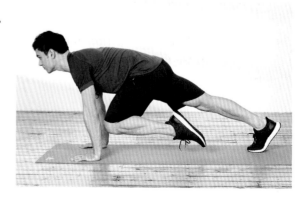

▶ Upward-facing Dog

This is the opposite of the Downward-facing Dog. Start in a press-up position and slowly drop your hips to the floor. Straighten your arms and lift your torso and upper legs a few inches off the floor. Open your chest and squeeze your legs and glutes to try and get your head as close to the sky as you can.

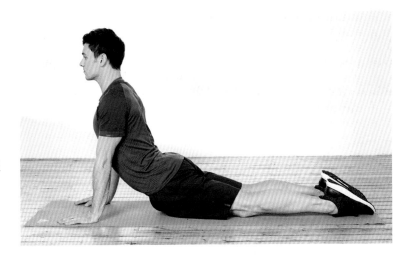

▶ Cat-Cow

1   Begin on your hands and knees with your wrists directly under your shoulders and your knees under your hips.

2   As you inhale, move into the 'Cow' pose by letting your stomach drop towards the mat. Lift your chin and chest and gaze towards the ceiling.

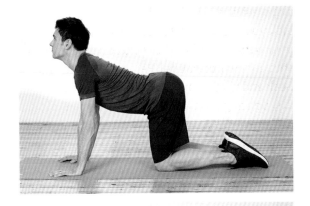

3   Then on your exhalation, move into the 'Cat' pose by drawing your stomach to your spine and rounding your back towards the ceiling. Release the crown of your head towards the floor but don't force your chin to your chest. This is a great way to mobilise your spine.

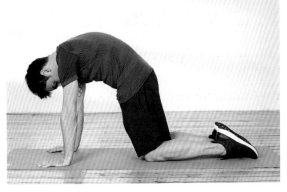

▶ Warrior 1

1 Stand with your feet hip distance apart and your arms at your sides. Step your feet wide apart (about 1–1.5 metres) and turn your right foot out 90 degrees. Pivot your left foot 45 degrees to the right so that your right heel is aligned with the arch of your left foot. Keep your pelvis towards the front of the mat. Press your weight through your left heel and bend your right knee over your right ankle.

2 Reach your arms up parallel or press your palms together. Look straight ahead or, if it's comfortable, gently tilt your head back and gaze up at your thumbs. To come out of the pose, press your left heel firmly into the mat and straighten your right knee. Turn your feet forward and release your arms. Repeat on the other side.

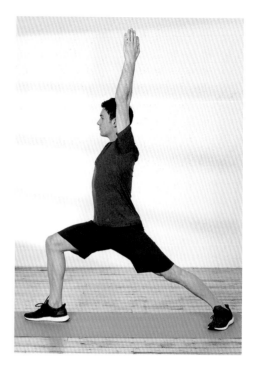

▼ Reverse Warrior

From Warrior 2, bring the left hand down to rest on the left leg. Stretch the right arm towards the ceiling. Place your left arm either behind your back or in front of your stomach, depending on your flexibility levels. Look straight ahead or at the ceiling. Keep the right knee bent and relax.

▼ Warrior 2

Follow the instructions for Warrior 1 but then open your arms out wide. Gently widen the stance and then turn both hip bones to face the side. Keep reaching out with your fingertips.

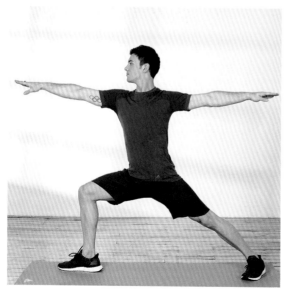

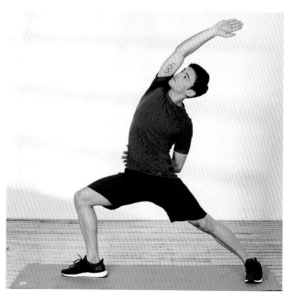

▶ Yoga Flow Press-ups

This is also known as a sun salutation. The aim is to flow between the movements, inhaling and exhaling between positions. Inhale: start in a plank position (1). Exhale: drop down into a press-up and hold just off the floor (2). Inhale: engage your glutes and push your hips to the floor, extending your arms and torso upwards so you finish in an Upward-facing Dog position (3). Exhale: push from there into a Downward-facing Dog (4). Inhale: return to a plank position (5). Repeat.

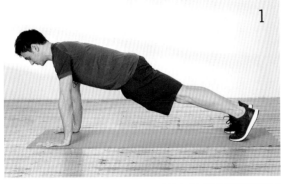

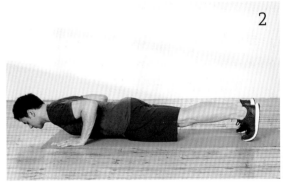

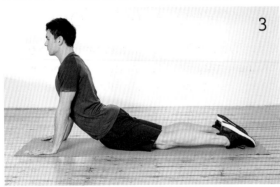

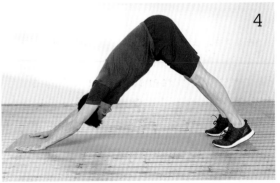

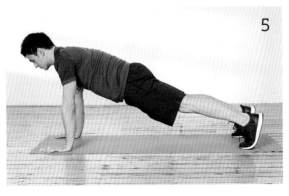

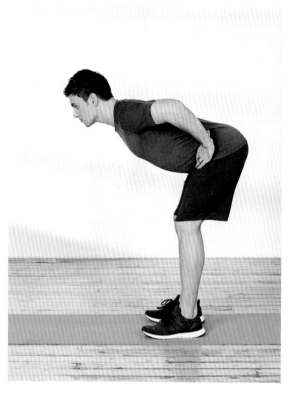 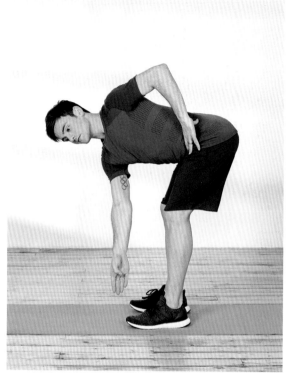

▶ RDL Twists

1 This is a great way to strengthen hamstrings, back and glutes. Stand straight with a slight bend in your knees. Keep your chest up and shoulders engaged (like grabbing a pencil between your shoulder blades).

2 Push your weight back into your heels and hinge forward at the hips until you can feel the stretch. Keep your shoulder blades back and your knees soft. Twist your whole torso, lifting your left shoulder up, and reach across with your right arm. Repeat on the other side with your right arm reaching across. Squeeze to come up.

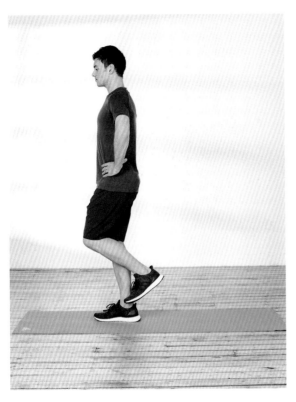
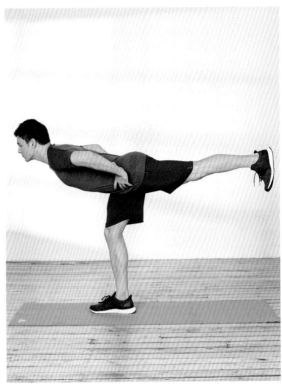

▶ Single Leg RDL

1   Stand with your feet shoulder width apart and knees slightly bent and raise one leg off the floor. Flex the knee on the supporting leg to about 15–20 degrees to activate the glutes.

2   Without changing the bend in your knee, hinge at your hips and lower your torso so it's almost parallel with the floor. Keep your torso in line with the back leg. Squeeze and raise your torso back to standing position.

Sumo Squat Touches

1 Place your feet significantly wider than hip distance apart. Turn your toes out by 45 degrees and hold your hands in front of you.

2 Lower yourself by bending your hips and knees. Keep your core tight and your back straight and do not let your knees move over your toes. Push up through your heels to standing and repeat. This is great for hip mobility.

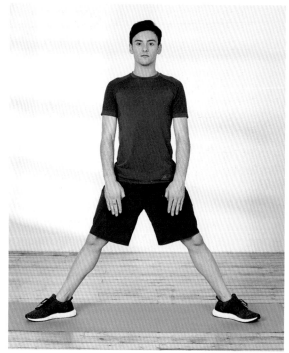

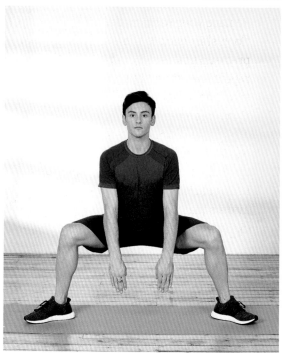

Gorilla Complex

Start in a standing position (1), then go into a forward fold (bend your knees slightly if necessary). Walk your hands out (2) to a press-up position, keeping your arms extended. From there bring your left leg outside your left hand (3), letting the opposite knee drop down towards the floor. Now take your left hand and reach it up towards the sky, opening up your chest, back and hips at the same time (4). Replace your hand on the floor, shift back to the press-up position (5) and repeat the movement, this time bringing your right leg forward and stretching your right arm up. Shift back to a press-up position, walk your hands back and move into a squat position (6). Extend one arm up straight (7), then the other arm, then stand up straight (8). Repeat.

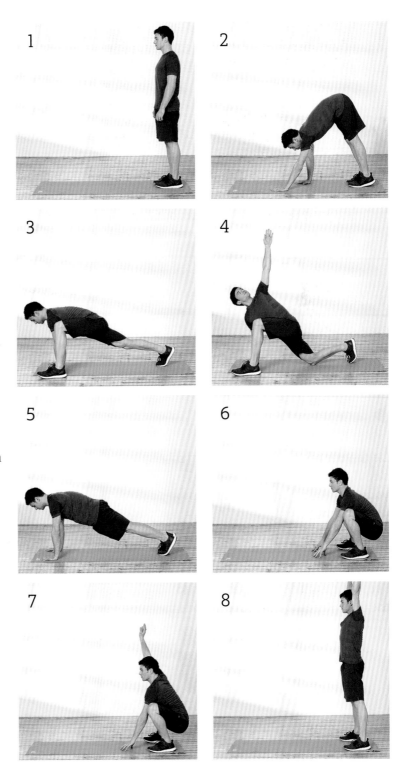

▶ Bird Dog

Go to four-point kneeling position with your shoulders and feet hip width apart. Then lift your leg and opposite arm off the ground at the same time and extend them out until they are parallel to the floor, without any rotation in the hip. Reach as far apart from each other as possible to elongate your spine. You are going to need balance for this one! Gently lower yourself back to your starting position and repeat with the opposite limbs.

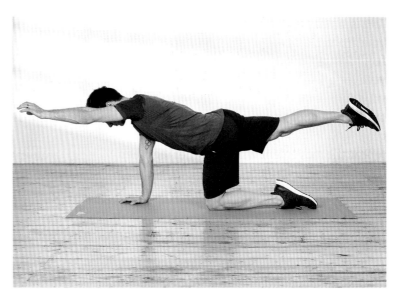

▶ Squat Circles

1 Squat down normally with your feet hip distance apart (1), shift your weight to one side (2), stand up with straight legs with your weight shifted to that side (3), go back to the centre (4) and then repeat on the other side.

2 Then do the movement in reverse: start in a standing position, push your weight to one side with straight legs, then squat down, keeping your weight on that side. Centralise at the bottom and then stand up.

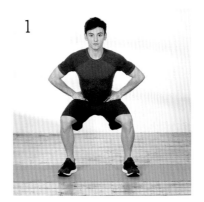

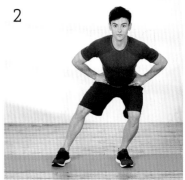

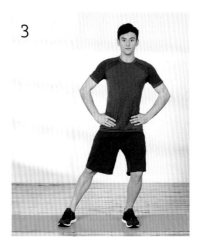

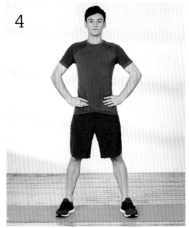

▶ Dead Bug Toe Taps

1. This exercise is similar to Bird Dog but this time you're lying on your back with your arms held up in front of you, pointing to the ceiling. Then bring your legs up so your knees are bent at 90-degree angles.

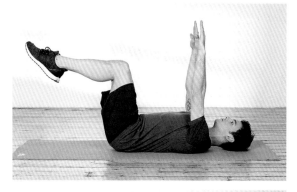

2. Slowly lower one leg and your opposite arm behind and away from you and straighten them, while keeping your lower back flat against the floor. If you feel your lower back lift, stop and don't go any further, that is your end range. Extend one leg and tap one toe to the floor. Repeat with the opposite leg.

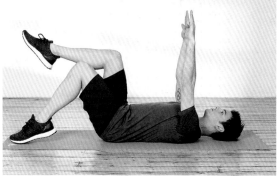

▶ Dead Bug Leg Extensions

With your knees at 90 degrees, extend one leg and stretch it away from you, down towards the floor, touching your calf and heel on the floor. Keep your back straight. Repeat with the opposite leg.

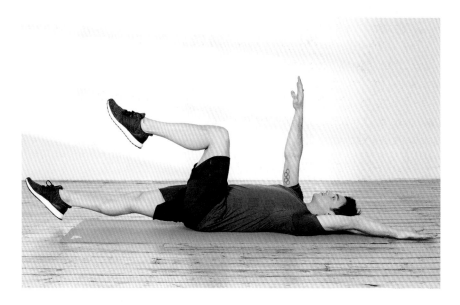

▶ Hip Bridges

Start by lying flat on your back with your knees bent and your arms by your hips. Tilt your pelvis upwards and push through your heels to slowly lift your hips while squeezing your glutes. It should feel like you are rolling your spine off the ground, one vertebra at a time. Try to create a diagonal line from your shoulders to your knees.

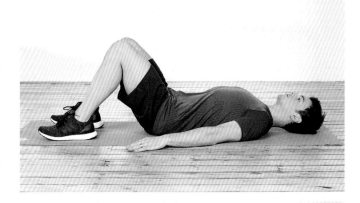

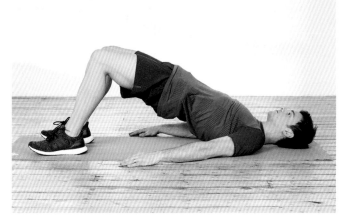

▶ Straight Leg Hip Bridges

At the top of the Hip Bridge, extend one leg out straight while keeping your hips level and engaging your core. Gently bring the leg back down and repeat on the other side.

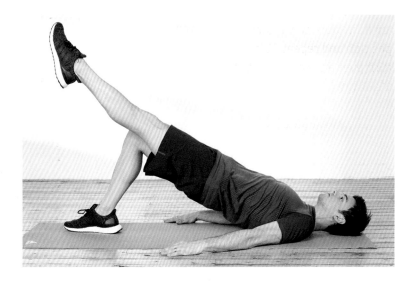

▶ Clams

1 Lie on your side with your knees bent at 90 degrees and your legs stacked on top of each other. Adjust your hips and torso so they are perpendicular to the floor.

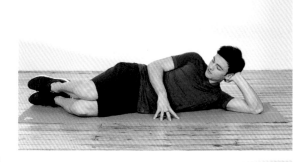

2 With your core engaged, rotate your top leg at the hip to bring your top knee upwards, like a clam. Stop before you feel your body rolling backwards. Return to the starting position and repeat. Then turn over and repeat on the other side.

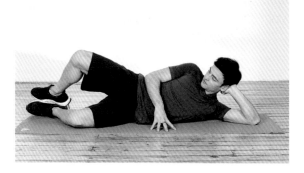

▶ Straight Leg Clams

Start in the same position as a clam but keep your top leg straight and extended with your body line. Keeping your stomach muscles tight and your top leg straight, lift the leg up. Return to the starting position and repeat. Then turn over and repeat on the other side.

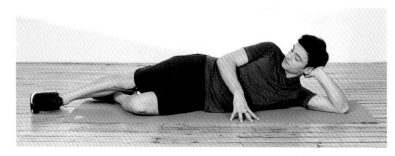

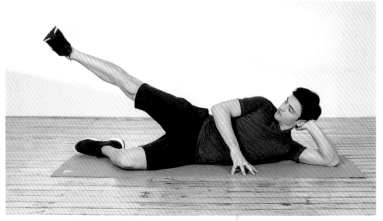

Plank Knee Twist

Start in a high plank position with your arms straight. Keep your back and bum straight. Bend one knee and twist it towards the opposite elbow. Repeat on your other side.

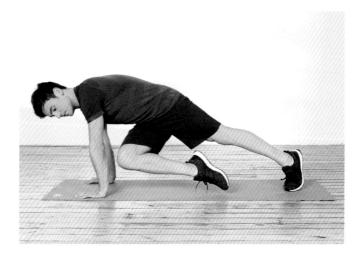

Kneeling Hip Flexor Stretch

1 Start from a kneeling position. Lift one knee up and place your foot slightly in front of your knee.

2 Exhale as you bend your front knee and lean forward. Hold the stretch, keeping your glutes squeezed and pelvis tilted underneath you to protect your back and maintain a good posture. Repeat the movement and then change sides.

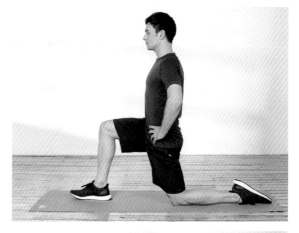

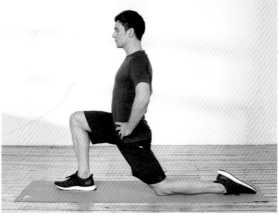

▶ Pigeon Pose

1 Start on all fours on your hands and knees. Bring your right knee forward and place it behind your right wrist. Place your ankle in front of your left hip. The more your lower leg is parallel with the front of your mat, the wider the stretch.

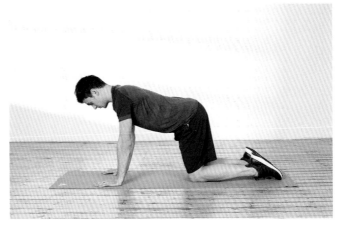

2 Slide your left leg back, straighten your knee and point your toes, with your heel pointing towards the ceiling. Lower yourself down and keep your hips level.

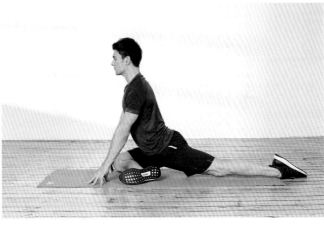

3 As you inhale, lift your upper body, come on to your fingertips with your hands shoulder width apart, draw your tummy in and open your chest. As you exhale, walk your hands forward on your fingertips and lower your upper body to the floor. To come out of the pose, push back through your fingers and lift your hips before moving back into all fours. Repeat with the other leg.

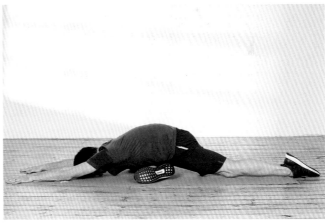

▶ Frog Stretch

This is a great stretch to release your hip flexors. Support yourself on your knees and forearms. Begin to take your knees out wider than your hips, then your feet out wider than your knees. Pull your hips back and press your pelvis down.

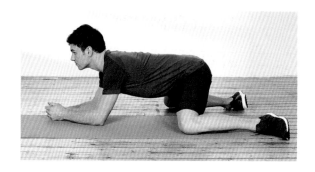

▼ Frog Stretch Rocks

Push your hips back and then rock forward and squeeze your glutes. To extend this further, push up on your hands.

▼ Side Plank Touches

Start on your side on one elbow. Raise your hips until your body is in a straight line from head to feet. Drop your hip to touch the floor if you can, or go as low as possible.

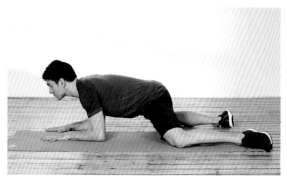

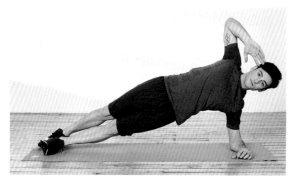

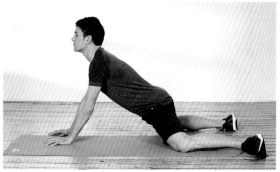

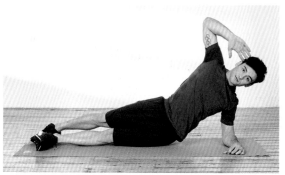

▶ Forward Fold

Hinge at the hips and let your hands dangle to the ground. Bend your legs slightly if needed and hang like a rag doll. You might find it easier to hold your arms at the elbow. Come up slowly.

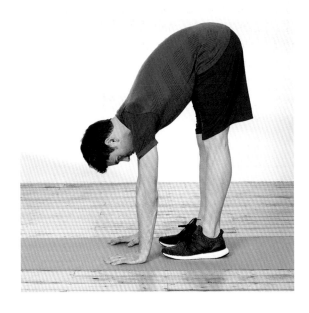

▶ Shoulder Extension

Kneel on the floor with straight arms resting on a bed, sofa or bench and push your chest towards the ground.

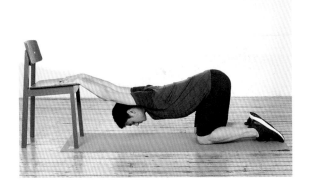

▶ Reverse Shoulder Extension

Face away from the bed, sofa or bench and place your hands narrow behind you with your palms facing away from you. Gently kneel or squat down to feel the stretch in the front of your shoulders.

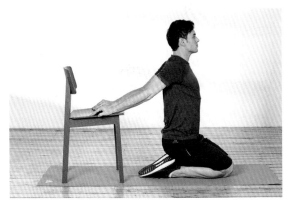

This workout is great for when you get out of bed and need to loosen up and get rid of any aches and pains. The Cat-Cow will start by loosening up your spine and opening up the chest, while the other exercises will target the major muscle groups and energise you for the day. It is also a good set of exercises to do as a mobility warm-up for more intense exercises afterwards. Follow your breath to move between repetitions and exercises.

WAKE-UP CALL WORKOUT

8 x

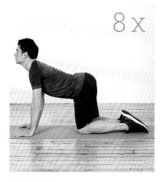

CAT-COW

8 x

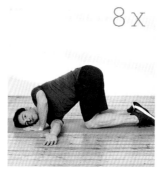

THREAD THE NEEDLE ON ONE SIDE, THEN 8 ON THE OTHER SIDE

8 x

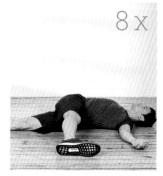

IRON CROSS ON EACH SIDE, ALTERNATING SIDES

8 x

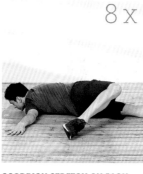

SCORPION STRETCH ON EACH SIDE, ALTERNATING SIDES

8 x

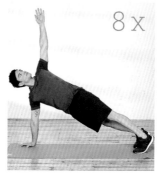

T PRESS-UPS ON EACH SIDE, ALTERNATING SIDES

8 x

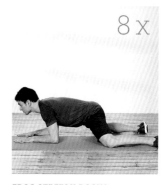

FROG STRETCH ROCKS

8 x

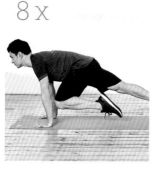

DOWNWARD-FACING DOG KNEE TUCKS ON EACH SIDE

8 x

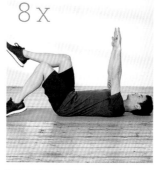

DEAD BUG TOE TAPS ON EACH SIDE, ALTERNATING SIDES

Beginners can follow the routine once, intermediates twice and advanced three times. This workout will engage your core muscles and all your major muscle groups. Lots of people ask me about how they can engage their lower abdominal muscles and these exercises are a great way to start. My top tip is to pull up your pelvic-floor muscles and try to keep them engaged throughout.

2.

STRENGTHEN, STRETCH & SCULPT WORKOUT

8 x
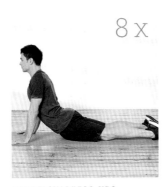
YOGA FLOW PRESS-UPS

8 x
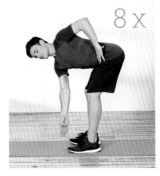
RDL TWISTS

8 x
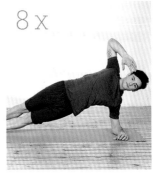
SIDE PLANK TOUCHES ON ONE SIDE, THEN 8 ON THE OTHER SIDE

8 x
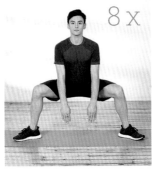
SUMO SQUAT TOUCHES

8 x
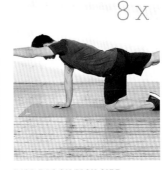
BIRD DOG ON EACH SIDE, ALTERNATING SIDES

8 x
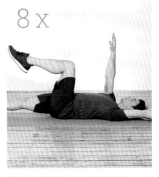
DEAD BUG LEG EXTENSIONS

8 x
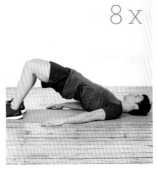
HIP BRIDGES

8 x
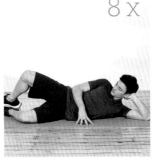
CLAMS ON ONE SIDE, THEN 8 ON THE OTHER SIDE

6.00

7.00

8.00 ◄ **8.00** A.M.

9.00

10.00

11.00

12.00

13.00

14.00

15.00

16.00

17.00

18.00

19.00

20.00

21.00

22.00

23.00

HABIT 2

POSITIVITY & MENTAL CARE

Ways you can start treating yourself better today!

It is very easy to be our own worst enemies and put our needs on the back-burner, which is why we end up frazzled, rundown and overwhelmed. Self-care is quite an individual thing but here are some ideas about the small things you can do to treat yourself better.

Take time to plan your day
So much of our time is spent running from A to B, with the idea that everything is taking too much time. Organise your day in a friendlier way. Of course, there will be times when you are unavoidably busy but try to carve out time each day to do something special that you enjoy, even if it's just having a bath or calling a friend. I factor in at least an hour each day to cook dinner and talk to my husband about how our days have been.

Let go of negative energy
When someone says something that annoys us or upsets us, it can be easy to go over and over it in our minds. Resist the urge to fight back and let go of negative energy. Try to show everyone kindness and compassion. Just because someone has made you feel a certain way, it doesn't mean it's right to try to make them feel that way too. It won't make either of you feel any better in the long run.

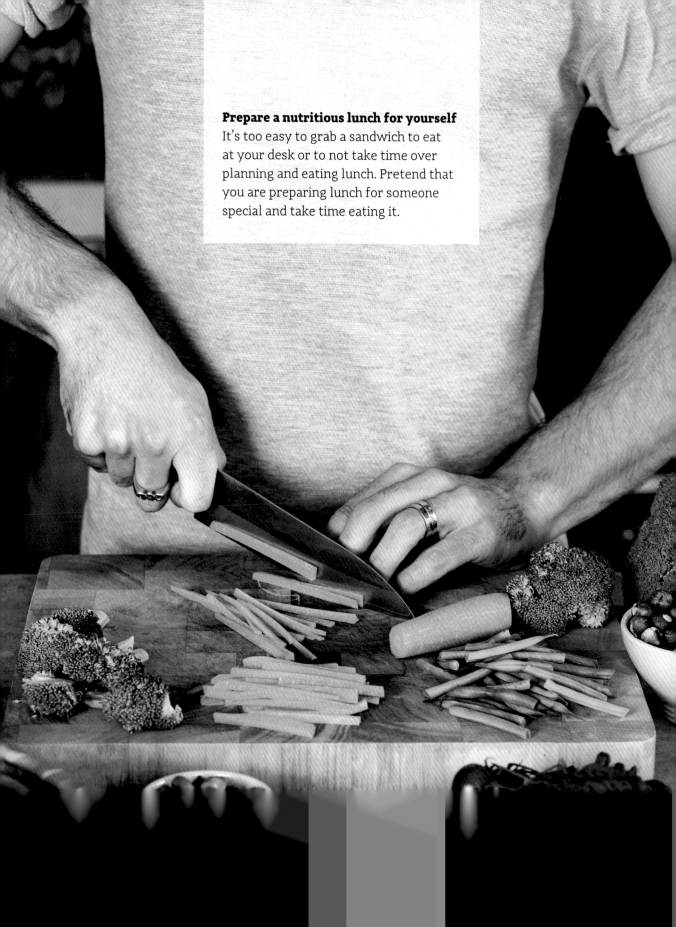

Prepare a nutritious lunch for yourself
It's too easy to grab a sandwich to eat at your desk or to not take time over planning and eating lunch. Pretend that you are preparing lunch for someone special and take time eating it.

Surround yourself with people who bring out the best in you

These are the people who make you laugh, inspire you to achieve your goals, or empower you to make positive changes. Whether this applies to family members, friends, partners, co-workers or acquaintances, these are the people you want to be spending your time with, rather than those who drain your energy or are negative.

Think about your own needs and how to meet them

Try to show the same kindness to yourself that you show to others and think about your own needs, whether emotional, physical or relationship-based. Research shows that recognising these needs is linked to better relationships and improved emotional stability.

Get outside

This is one of the simplest things we can do to boost our mental and physical health. Among other proven scientific benefits, research suggests that being outside in nature restores mental energy, boosts immunity, improves memory, relieves stress, reduces inflammation and improves concentration. Consider working out in the great outdoors – this has been shown to relieve depression, decrease tension and boost mental health.

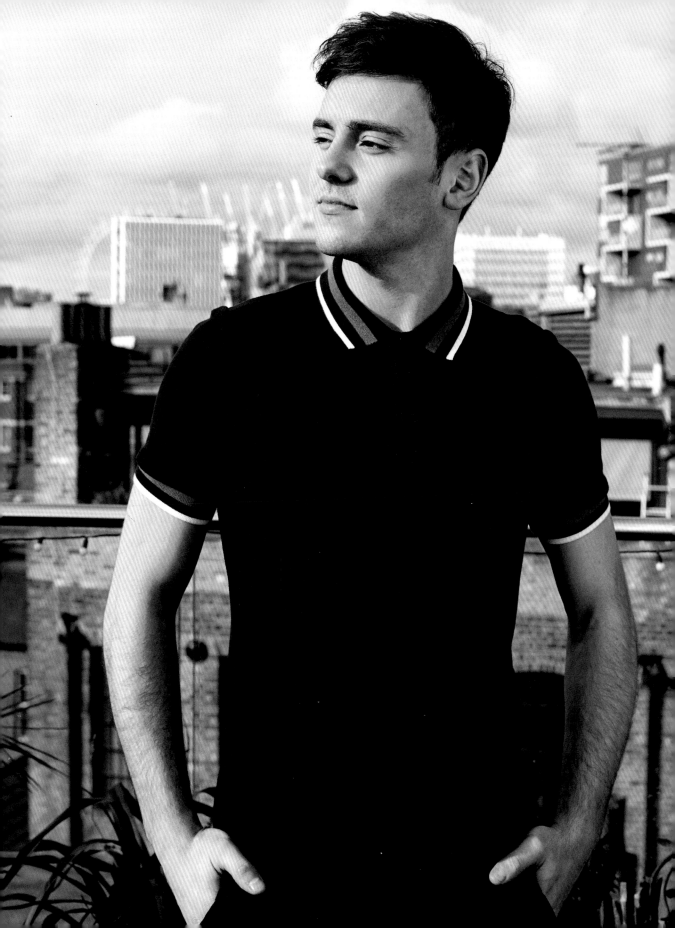

3 exercises to breathe yourself calm

Have you ever noticed that when you take a deliberately deep breath, you feel super-relaxed? Breathwork is a general term for breathing exercises that can improve mental, physical and spiritual health. Drawn from Eastern practices like yoga and tai chi, it encourages controlled breathing to keep your body and mind functioning at their best and will promote feelings of calm and relaxation. Many experts suggest that focusing on breathing brings increased self-awareness and mindfulness.

Equal breathing: This equal-ratio breathing technique is practised by making sure that the inhalation is the same length as the exhalation. To start, inhale for the count of four and exhale for the count of four, all through the nose. This is said to be soothing and helps to calm the mind. You can do this any time, in any place.

2

Abdominal breathing technique: With one hand on your tummy and the other on your chest, inhale to feel your diaphragm inflate with enough air to stretch the lungs. Exhale slowly. The slower you breathe, the quieter your mind will become. Aim to take deep and steady breaths for ten minutes.

4-7-8 breathing: This exercise – also referred to as 'The Relaxing Breath', is based on pranayama, an ancient Indian practice that means 'regulation of breath'. It's done by first exhaling through the mouth, making a 'whooshing' noise. Close your mouth and inhale quietly for a count of four. Then hold your breath for a count of seven. Then exhale completely through your mouth for a count of eight, making a whooshing noise. Inhale again and repeat the cycle at least five more times. Breathing out for so long can feel hard to achieve at times – and you might pull some weird faces, but the benefits are worth it! I always try and do this after a workout because it automatically clicks my body into recovery mode, stimulating the parasympathetic nervous system. This allows the body to recover from the stress of the workout and diverts more blood to the digestive tract, allowing for better nutrient transportation around the body.

Top tips to beat the Sunday-night blues

One minute you are having a brilliant weekend, then the next moment it's Sunday night and you are overcome by waves of dread about the enormity of the week ahead. Even if you love what you do, Sunday nights can feel tough; apparently two-thirds of us experience the phenomenon known as 'Sunday-night blues'. Sunday is my day off but I always feel like Sunday night comes round too quickly! Here are some things you can do to try and ward off these feelings.

Schedule fun plans for Sunday instead of Saturday

Try and distract yourself by planning a meal with friends on Sunday, rather than Saturday. It doesn't have to be a late night but will keep you in weekend mode for a few hours longer.

Get organised

Instead of heading straight to the sofa for a Netflix marathon, use the time to get organised for the week ahead, so you are less stressed about your to-do list and more positive by the time Monday rolls round. Preparing nutritious meals and snacks in advance will not only help you save money but will make you feel good too.

Recognise the feeling!

Recognise that many other people also feel the same way on a Sunday evening and that it will soon be over. Like many other things, it's just a temporary feeling and soon Friday will roll around again!

Avoid Saturday night blowouts

Alcohol has many effects on the mind and body and is most notably a depressant. With a hangover, the reason you feel so sad and sluggish is because the levels of dopamine (the 'pleasure' chemical) in your body are really depleted. Some people are more affected than others, but it will eventually catch up with you!

Avoid the temptation to catch up on sleep

Experts say you can get too much sleep and long lie-ins can create what they call 'social jet lag' – where our body clocks are out of kilter. This affects our natural rhythms, making us feel worse and less rested. For me, more than nine hours can make me feel lethargic and out of sync. Sometimes I will go to bed an hour later and get up an hour later but any more than this and I don't feel good!

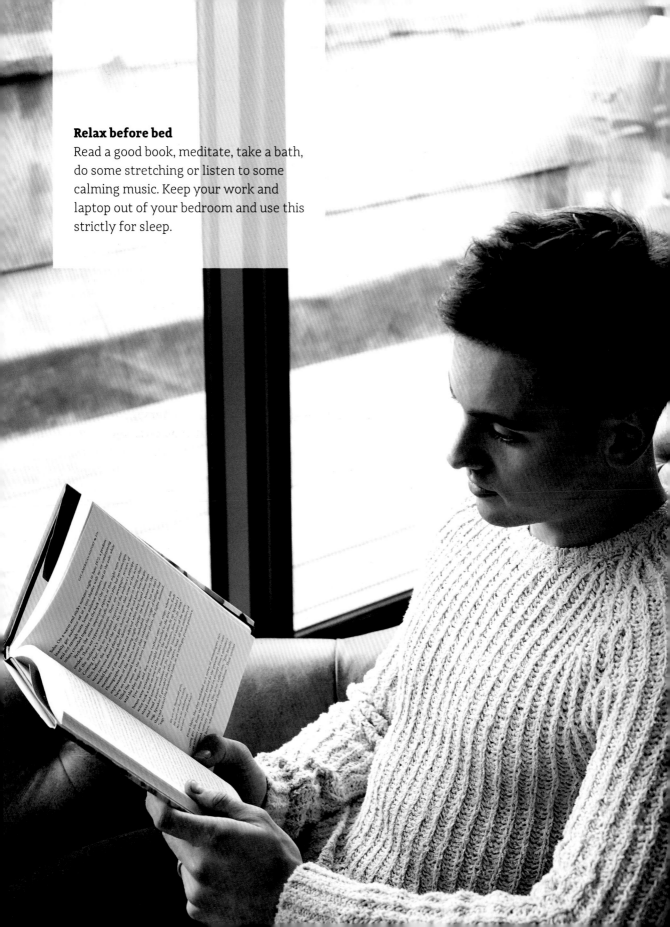

Relax before bed

Read a good book, meditate, take a bath, do some stretching or listen to some calming music. Keep your work and laptop out of your bedroom and use this strictly for sleep.

6.00

7.00

8.00

9.00 ◀ **9.00** A.M.

10.00

11.00

12.00

13.00

14.00

15.00

16.00

17.00

18.00

19.00

20.00

21.00

22.00

23.00

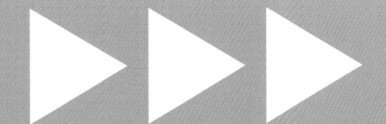

HABIT 3
IMMUNE
SYSTEM

Having always been health-conscious, I am lucky because I generally don't suffer from coughs and colds. But I'm not completely immune and from time to time, I'll have cold symptoms, bouts of tiredness and feel under the weather. This can be a disaster for training and competitions. The last thing I need as I'm standing on the end of a board is a runny nose or tickly throat! But for many of us, it's exactly during those times when we really could do without being ill, that we are struck down by a cold or other illness. Most areas of our health and well-being can be controlled by forming a few extra habits that will prevent – or at the very least reduce – illnesses and other problems. So what can you do to boost your immunity?

The immune system is our bodies' natural defence against illness and on the whole, it does a remarkable job of protecting us from disease-causing microorganisms. It is an interactive network of organs, antibodies, white blood cells, proteins and other chemicals that recognise foreign bodies like bacteria and viruses from the body's normal healthy tissues and destroy them. However, it doesn't always protect us from the barrage of germs we come into contact with and some will invade successfully, making us sick. Having a healthy immune system does not mean that we won't get a cold but it will mean our ability to fight it off quicker is stronger, which may mean the difference between a sniffle and a full-on cold. It is important to note that our immune system is complex; because it is not a single entity but a system, it relies on many different things and therefore requires balance and harmony. Sometimes our immune system can malfunction, causing illnesses such as autoimmune diseases and allergies. I suffer from hay fever over the spring and summer months, so always ensure I get a healthy dose of vitamins (especially vitamin C, which is said to be a natural antihistamine) when I feel my nose start to itch and my eyes water. You may just think about boosting immunity during the winter months but our immune systems work hard all year round and an infection can happen at any time. Stress and immunity are intrinsically linked and studies have shown that stress can play havoc with our bodies and leave us more susceptible to becoming ill, so being more mindful and practising some of the other habits in this book will help.

Hand washing is also an important tool in the fight against germs. In London, for example, an estimated 2.29 billion people use the buses and 1.34 billion use the Underground every year, making it a hotbed for germs and bacteria. Metal poles, seats, tray tables and other surfaces are often contaminated with microbes and bacteria. Keeping our hands clean is one of the most important steps we can take to avoid illnesses and spreading germs, so if you travel to work by public transport, make sure you wash your hands when you get there. This might seem an inconvenience, but washing your hands for 20 seconds is far less annoying than spending two weeks in bed with the flu. Always ensure you wash your hands properly with soap and water, using the water first, then lathering your hands in soap and rubbing and washing every area, including the backs of your fingers. I read recently about washing them for the time it takes to sing 'Happy Birthday' twice – around 20 seconds – to fully get rid of germs. It's also really important to dry your hands properly because research shows that bacteria tend to spread faster on damp or wet hands. I also carry hand sanitiser around with me. Try to remember to wash your hands several times a day and always before you eat. Also, don't forget to clean your mobile phone from time to time – according to research, our phones are ten times dirtier than most toilet seats! Yikes!

IF YOU DO ONE THING ...
Wash your hands thoroughly for 20 seconds using soap and water after travelling on public transport.

6 ways to boost

We all know what it feels like to have a cold coming on: headache, painful sinuses and a tickly throat. Here are some sure-fire ways to boost your immunity with these germ-zappers.

1

Eat a nutrient-packed diet: The old-fashioned ways of keeping our immune systems healthy through diet and exercise really do work. A varied diet of fruit, vegetables, whole grains and lean proteins will help your body defend itself against germs. Avoid reaching for junk food when you start to feel unwell; in particular, polyunsaturated fats tend to supress our immune systems. One of the first things I do when I start to feel ill is to increase my vitamin C intake, eating lots of fruits and vegetables.

2

Recruit an exercise buddy: Working out will not only keep your waist trim but it has been proven that people with more sedentary lifestyles are far more likely to get colds and other infectious diseases. Working out with an exercise buddy will not only help you achieve your fitness goals but will make you work harder and keep you motivated.

3

Get enough sleep: When life is busy it can feel like the best way to get everything done on your to-do list is to cut down on sleep. However, not prioritising sleep can have disastrous health consequences. Sleep deprivation and stress increase the production of the hormone cortisol, prolonged elevation of which can suppress our immune function. Poor sleep is also associated with reduced numbers of the cells that fight germs.

your immunity

4

Eat probiotic foods: Did you know that around 70 per cent of your immunity is in your gut? There are trillions of beneficial bacteria located here that will help you absorb nutrients and fight off infections. Recent research shows that eating food live with active cultures may offer additional benefits compared to regular foods. Good examples include live yoghurt, kefir and cultured vegetables like sauerkraut and kimchi.

5

Cut down your meat intake: Plant-based diets are naturally anti-inflammatory because they are high in fibre, antioxidants and other nutrients and much lower in inflammatory triggers like saturated fats. Studies have shown that people who do not eat meat and follow plant-based diets reduce their levels of C-reactive protein, an indication of inflammation in their body. Aim to have meat-free days at least three days per week if possible.

6

Catch some rays: Sunlight triggers the skin's production of vitamin D and this will boost your immune system. Don't get cooped up: when the sun is shining, get outside and enjoy it! In the summer months, you can be without sunscreen for 20 minutes, although always remember to apply it generously if you will be outside longer, especially to your face. As well as the health risks, sun damage will be the fastest thing to age you, so protect those pretty little faces.

Top inflammation-fighting foods and how to incorporate them into your diet

Inflammation is a bodily function that is not always bad because without it we can't heal. When the body is ill or injured the lymphatic or immune system gets to work, bringing an army of white blood cells to the problem area. In a healthy body, inflammation is a normal and effective response that will facilitate healing. However, when the immune system overreaches and begins attacking healthy tissues, this results in autoimmune disorders. For example, asthma creates inflamed airways and inflammation related to diabetes results in insulin resistance. There are certain foods that we can incorporate into our diet to reduce inflammation.

Fatty fish

Oily fish like tuna, salmon, mackerel and sardines are high in omega-3 fatty acids, which can help to reduce inflammation. Aim to eat fish once or twice a week, starting with tuna, if you are new to oily fish. Find healthy ways to eat oily fish, on its own or in salads.

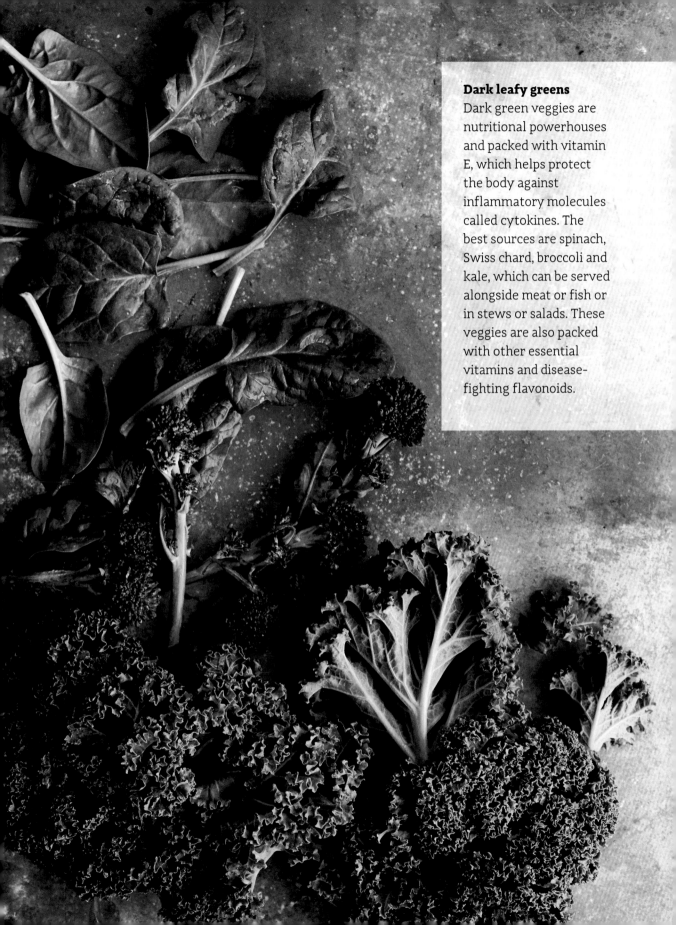

Dark leafy greens

Dark green veggies are nutritional powerhouses and packed with vitamin E, which helps protect the body against inflammatory molecules called cytokines. The best sources are spinach, Swiss chard, broccoli and kale, which can be served alongside meat or fish or in stews or salads. These veggies are also packed with other essential vitamins and disease-fighting flavonoids.

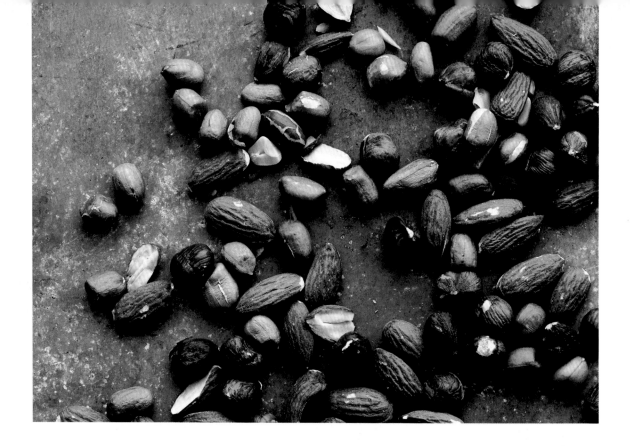

Nuts

Healthy nuts are packed with polyunsaturated and monounsaturated fats and have major anti-inflammatory effects. In particular, almonds, hazelnuts, pecan nuts and peanuts are excellent sources of vitamin E. They are great for snacks, sprinkled on porridge or salads or enjoyed as nut butters.

Extra virgin olive oil

The Mediterranean diet is famous for lowering the risk of chronic disease. Olive oil is said to be one of the most important parts of this diet because it contains nutrients called polyphenols, which stop the release of inflammatory compounds. Extra virgin olive oil contains the most antioxidants and has fewer chemicals than standard olive oil. If your recipe calls for canola oil or vegetable oil, substitute these for extra virgin olive oil; this can make a real difference.

Tomatoes

High in vitamin C, potassium and lycopene, an antioxidant known for its anti-inflammatory properties, tomatoes are a must-have on your shopping list. Cooked tomatoes contain even more lycopene than raw ones, so say yes to tomato sauce – homemade, of course!

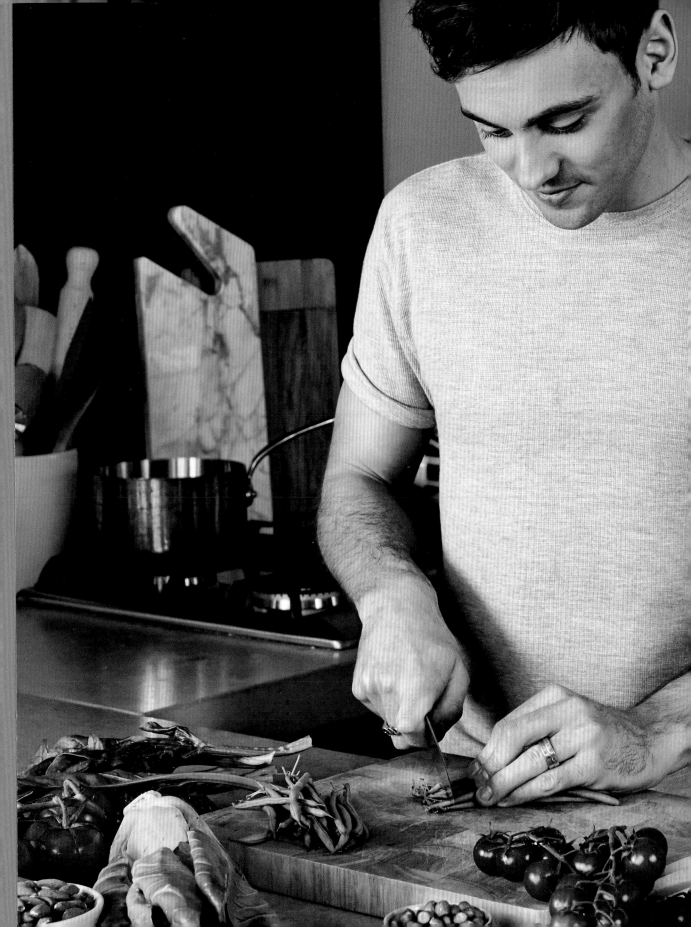

6.00

7.00

8.00

9.00

10.00

11.00

12.00

13.00 ◄ **1.00** P.M.

14.00

15.00

16.00

17.00

18.00

19.00

20.00

21.00

22.00

23.00

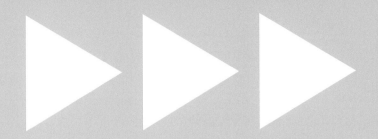

HABIT 4
FOOD

Cooking at home can really kick-start a healthy lifestyle. You can discover new recipes, learn about food, create and stick to a meal plan and be inspired to live a healthier life. When people talk about not having time to cook from scratch, I understand. When you've had a busy day the last thing you might feel like doing is spending half an hour cooking a meal. In the mornings, it can feel even easier to not prepare food for lunch if you are in a rush to leave the house and are surrounded by easy, takeaway options near your workplace. However, there is a simple solution – it just involves a bit of planning! Cooking in the evening doesn't need to be laborious and home-cooked meals bring with them a raft of benefits. All my dishes in this book contain ingredients you are likely to have in your cupboard or are easy to shop for and many of the recipes take less than 15 minutes to prepare. If you make double of every dinner, or batch-cook a few portions, you will always have a fresh and healthy lunch to hand. I've also included some recipes that you can tweak to make a fresh option for lunch, so you don't feel like you are eating the same dish twice.

There has been a lot of talk in recent years about 'clean eating' but for me this concept is simple; the more we can cook from scratch so we know exactly what goes into our food, the better. Many commercially prepared foods are high in salt, fat and sugar. And you don't know exactly what goes into them (as an example, McDonald's fries have 19 ingredients!). By cooking your meals yourself, you can choose to steam or grill foods rather than fry them, helping to reduce fat and preserve more of their nutritional value. It also allows you to balance both portion size and the amount of protein, carbohydrate and fat you are getting each day, plus all the essential vitamins and minerals you need. By doing this, you are more likely to have a productive afternoon working and less likely to have a mid-afternoon slump and reach for the biscuit tin! You won't just be eating better but you will save money too; if you spend about £5 a day now, you will save over £100 per month.

Far from being a chore, cooking is a really great way to switch off after a busy day. I love the creative side of cooking – there are no rights and wrongs. I love experimenting with food and I find the process really absorbing and relaxing. One thing I love to do for Lance is just see what we have in the fridge and cupboards and make something up! My mum used to call it 'if-it's' – as in 'if it's there and it's not out of date, go for it!' It was her way of pulling together all the ingredients we hadn't used to make something delicious out of them. Try to do your own 'if-it's' challenge and see what you can create!

All the recipe suggestions in this book are packed full of veggies – some contain fish and meat as well, while others are strictly vegan. We have aimed to make it simple to navigate, with symbols to show vegetarian recipes, vegan recipes, recipes which contain fish and those that only need one pan (for those days when you can't face mountains of washing-up!). All the ingredients are easy to get hold of, so there shouldn't be any waste. Some recipes are for four people or more (so ideal to save for lunch if you are just cooking for two) but most serve one or two and can be easily doubled or trebled if you are cooking for a crowd, or planning a whole week's lunches in advance. You'll find all the nutritional breakdowns on pages 186–9. Happy cooking!

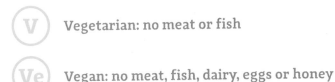

(V) Vegetarian: no meat or fish

(Ve) Vegan: no meat, fish, dairy, eggs or honey

Fish/seafood: includes these nutritional powerhouses

One pan: to reduce washing-up!

IF YOU DO ONE THING ...

Try to take a home-cooked lunch with you into work. Make double of every dinner you cook so you always have something fresh and healthy for lunch the next day.

5 ways to reset your relationship with food

1

Use neutral language: Avoid labelling foods as 'good', 'bad' or 'clean'. If you remove these words, then you take away negative feelings associated with eating 'banned' foods. If we completely ban sugar, for example, this often leads us to not having any and then bingeing. Adjust your mindset and adopt a more neutral approach.

2

Listen to your body: Every person is individual with different nutritional needs so instead of trying to eat a certain number of calories or beating yourself up when the scales show you have put on weight, tune into your body. Look inwards to decide how, when and what to eat. Eat when you are hungry and stop when you are full. Measure your weight and fitness progress by how you feel and how well your clothes fit.

PAY ATTENTION TO HOW DIFFERENT FOODS AFFECT YOUR EMOTIONS: DO CERTAIN THINGS INFLUENCE YOUR MOOD? MAKE A NOTE

How would you describe your relationship with food? How do you feel about your diet and the food you eat? Eating should always feel like a positive experience and listening to cues for hunger and developing healthy food habits that work with our bodies is key to our health and well-being.

3

Stop comparing yourself to others: So many people follow fad diets that promise quick and easy results. However, in the long term this is not a realistic approach to food and diet because invariably the weight they have lost goes back on. You need to find out what works for you and to stick to it.

4

Make friends with fat: Our bodies need fat to function properly and getting some healthy fats from natural sources in your diet is essential to good health. Good fats ensure we have sustained energy, so we are less likely to snack on refined carbohydrates and sugar. Good examples are eggs, nuts and avocados.

5

Give yourself permission to enjoy cooking and eating: Make time to cook, eat, sit down at the table with friends or family and enjoy the experience. Think about how the food nourishes your body.

Switch on your power foods

When life is busy with deadlines and stress, it is crucial to not reach for stodge and comfort foods. By eating some of the right foods, you can avoid rubbish moods, weight gains and constant colds. Here are some food superheroes to turn to.

Quinoa

Gluten-free, high in protein and one of the few plant foods that contains all the essential amino acids, quinoa packs a real punch. It also contains manganese that impacts hormones and digestive enzymes, making it easier for the body to digest and use the food you eat efficiently.

Chillies

Capsaicin, the compound that gives chillies their fiery flavour, boosts antibody-producing cells in our bodies by almost three times, according to one Korean University study. Chillies are also a great source of vitamin C, folic acid, manganese, beta-carotenes and other minerals.

Kale

As well as being packed with a host of antioxidants, kale is a great source of vitamin A, which promotes eye and skin health and vitamin B6, which helps maintain a healthy nervous and immune system. It's also a good source of fibre and one cup has almost as much vitamin C as an orange. I love kale leaves baked with just a drizzle of olive oil, as an alternative to crisps!

Green tea

This is my go-to choice when I want a hot drink with less caffeine than coffee or tea. Green tea is packed full of powerful antioxidants called polyphenols, which help to damage-proof the body, protecting its cells from toxins, ageing and disease. It can also improve cholesterol levels and reduce the risk of both heart disease and inflammation.

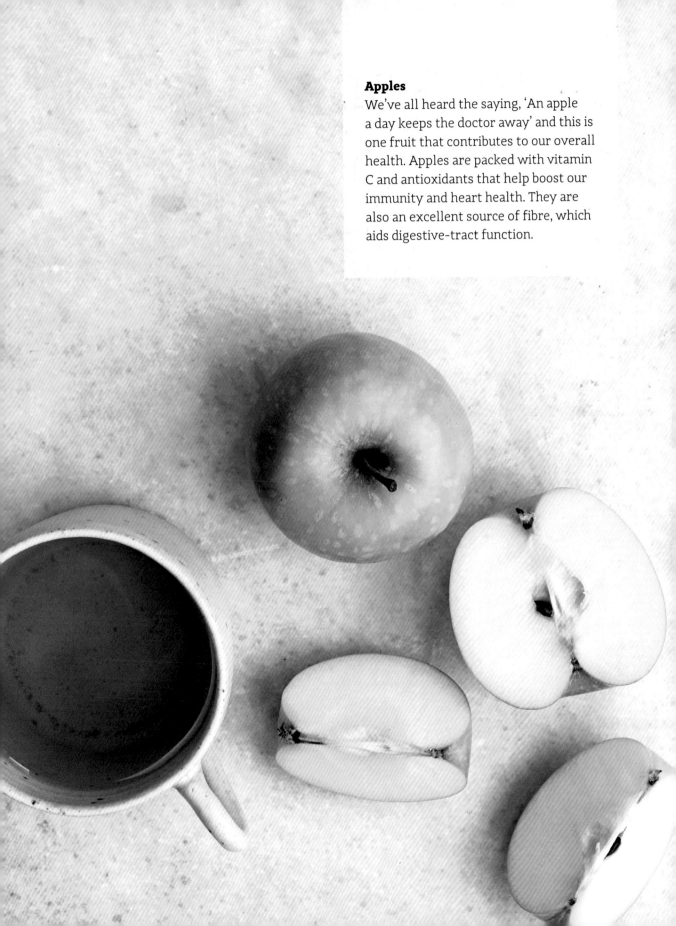

Apples

We've all heard the saying, 'An apple a day keeps the doctor away' and this is one fruit that contributes to our overall health. Apples are packed with vitamin C and antioxidants that help boost our immunity and heart health. They are also an excellent source of fibre, which aids digestive-tract function.

Tired all the time? Nutrition myths that are sapping your energy

What you put into your body will definitely determine how you feel but sometimes there is confusion about what is good and what isn't good for you. If you feel constantly tired, your diet may be to blame. Here are some truths you need to know:

Myth: cereal and breakfast drinks are a good choice
Truth: while pre-packaged cereal and breakfast drinks and instant porridge are a good source of fibre, protein and dairy, they are usually high in sugar. Some contain as much as 25g (6 teaspoons) of sugar per serving, which is your recommended amount of sugar in just one portion! The same applies to energy drinks; these are also often loaded with sugar and caffeine, so they will cause an energy rush and then a crash.

Myth: low-calorie foods are the best choice
Truth: when you want to make the right food choices, the low-fat and low-calorie option might seem best. However, many of these foods contain additives to increase their shelf life and give them a certain taste. Aim to eat plenty of food with a low glycaemic index (GI), so you keep your blood-sugar levels steady.

Myth: don't eat after 8 p.m.
Truth: obviously if you spend all evening grazing on biscuits while in front of the TV, that's not going to help you lose weight and feel good, but if you get home late, it is fine to eat a moderately sized, balanced meal for dinner. Calories are calories whatever time of the day you eat them!

Myth: all food labelled as 'natural' is good for you

Truth: beware of misleading food labels! Even products that are labelled as 'all natural' can be highly processed and contain high levels of sweeteners, like corn syrup and fructose. Many contain natural colourings and flavourings, which are made using the same chemical processes and are very similar to their artificial counterparts.

Myth: don't snack between meals

Truth: most people only need breakfast, lunch and dinner but if you've exercised, it's important to have a snack within 20 minutes of working out to replace energy stores and help with muscle repair. Make sure it contains protein and carbohydrates; my snacks of choice are protein shakes, Greek yoghurt, a protein bar or homemade protein balls!

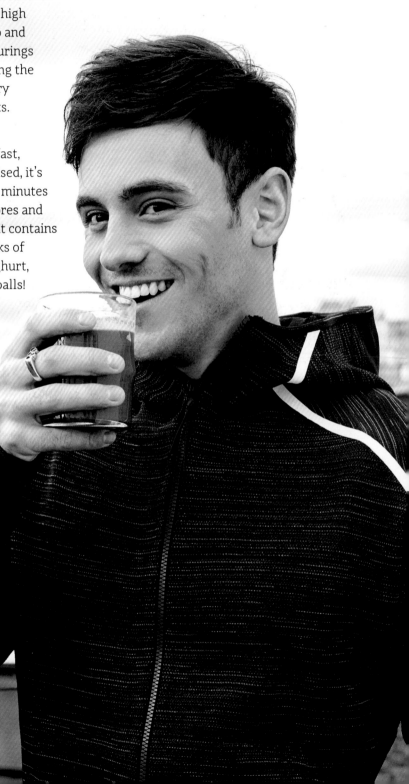

breakfasts

Start your day right with one of these
nutritious breakfasts, which include porridge,
muesli, eggs – and everything in between!
They are packed with protein and will fuel
you throughout your morning.

Smoky beans in a bun

Homemade beans are so much nicer than the canned version and are actually very quick to make from just a handful of ingredients. These ones are made in one pan with a paprika sauce, giving them a smoky and creamy taste.

SERVES 2 | PLUS 2 PORTIONS TO FREEZE
231 calories per serving

1 tbsp olive oil

½ red onion, finely chopped or grated

1 mild red chilli, deseeded and diced

1 tsp smoked paprika

200g canned chopped tomatoes

1 tsp tomato purée

400g can mixed beans, drained

70g bag of rocket

2 small ciabatta rolls (about 80g each)

sea salt and freshly ground black pepper

1 Heat 2 teaspoons of the oil in a frying pan over a medium heat. Stir in the red onion, chilli and 1 tablespoon of water and cook for 5–6 minutes.

2 Stir in the smoked paprika and cook for 1 minute. Add the chopped tomatoes, tomato purée and 200ml water and season well. Bring to a simmer and cook over a medium heat for 5 minutes. Stir in the beans and cook for a further 3–4 minutes until heated through.

3 Spoon half the beans into a sealable container and set aside.

4 To serve two people, toast the ciabatta rolls while you finely chop half the rocket. Stir the chopped rocket into the beans and season to taste. Put the ciabatta rolls on to two plates and spoon the remaining beans on to the base of each bun. Top with the remaining rocket, drizzle each with half the remaining olive oil and then add the ciabatta lids.

TOM'S TIP
Store the extra portions in the fridge for up to 4 days or in the freezer for up to a month.

Smoked salmon & courgette breakfast pots

Kick-start your day with this protein-rich brekkie, which is very simple to rustle up. I line ramekins with smoked salmon, then fill with a mixture of egg, cottage cheese, grated courgette and parsley. They are then just baked in the oven until set. This little pot will keep you feeling full for hours!

SERVES 2
318 calories per serving

120g smoked salmon slices

1 small courgette (about 125g)

2 large eggs

10g chopped parsley

3 tbsp cottage cheese

sea salt and freshly ground black pepper

To serve

2 small slices of wholemeal bread

6 cherry tomatoes, quartered

1 Preheat the oven to 200°C/180°C Fan/Gas 6.

2 Line two large, deep ramekins with the smoked salmon, so the base and sides are covered.

3 Grate the courgette using a coarse grater and put into a large bowl. Crack in the eggs, add the chopped parsley and cottage cheese and season well with salt and pepper. Use a fork to break up the eggs, then mix all the ingredients together.

4 Divide evenly between the ramekins and bake in the oven for 20–25 minutes, or until the filling has set.

5 Toast and halve the bread and arrange on two plates with the cherry tomatoes spooned on top. Season well and serve with the smoked salmon pots.

TOM'S TIP
These make a great, super-quick supper, too – in fact, if you're putting the oven on anyway, they would be great with a jacket potato, too. Just choose a spud that's as small as your fist and steam a couple of florets of broccoli to serve alongside.

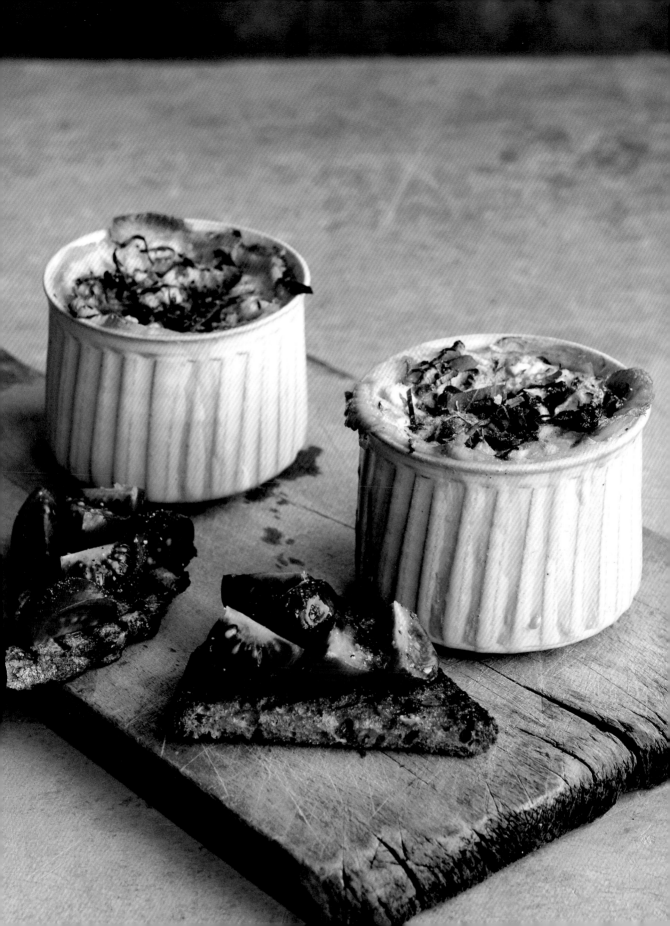

Tom's extra special slow-cooked eggs

This is the breakfast Lance and I make when we fancy a treat. It's really rich and filling so isn't something we enjoy every day but we love to make it at the weekend for brunch. Cooking the eggs with crème fraîche and milk, over a low heat, keeps them soft and creamy.

SERVES 2
394 calories per serving

4 large eggs

2 tbsp crème fraîche

2 tbsp milk

2 slices of sourdough or rye bread

4 slices of Parma ham

truffle oil

sea salt and freshly ground black pepper

1 Beat the eggs in a bowl then stir in the crème fraîche, milk and a good pinch of salt.

2 Pour into a medium pan and cook over a very low heat for about 3 minutes, or until the eggs are cooked but the mixture looks lovely and creamy. You can carry on cooking for longer if you prefer, but the longer you cook, the firmer the texture.

3 Toast the bread and put on to two plates. Spoon the slow-cooked eggs on top. Fold each slice of ham into a curl, placing two on top of each plate of eggs, then drizzle with the truffle oil. Season with black pepper and serve at once.

TOM'S TIP
This really is filling enough as it is, but if you fancy some spinach, add a big handful of baby leaves on the side or wilt them in a pan with a splash of water.

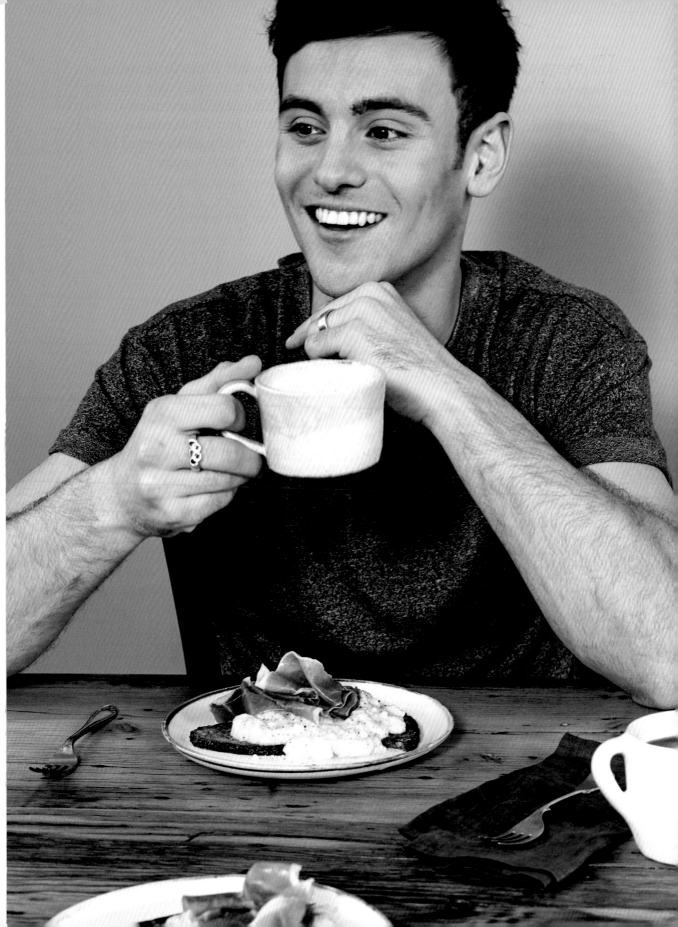

Sweetcorn pancakes

I've given the humble pancake a savoury twist by adding sweetcorn and spring onions. Using ground almonds makes them gluten-free and injects a dose of protein, monounsaturated fats and minerals like manganese, which helps the body form strong bones and regulates blood sugar. Serve with grilled tomatoes and crisp Parma ham on the side.

SERVES 2
266 calories per serving

For the pancakes

2 spring onions, finely chopped

1 corn on the cob, kernels sliced off (about 125g)

1 large egg

2 tbsp ground almonds

1^1/$_2$ tsp olive oil

sea salt and freshly ground black pepper

To serve

4 slices of Parma ham

2 vine tomatoes, halved through the middle

1 sprig of thyme

1 Preheat the grill.

2 Put the spring onions, sweetcorn kernels, egg and ground almonds into a bowl. Season well and beat everything together with a fork.

3 Arrange the Parma ham slices on a baking sheet and put the tomatoes alongside. Pick the leaves from the thyme sprig and sprinkle over the top of the tomatoes and season with black pepper. Grill until the Parma ham is crisp and the tomatoes have warmed through.

4 Meanwhile heat the oil in a large frying pan. Roughly portion the pancake mixture into four and once the oil is hot, spoon each of the four mounds into the pan, spaced well apart. Flatten them down slightly and cook until golden, around 1–2 minutes, then flip over and cook until golden on the other side.

5 Divide the Parma ham and tomatoes between two plates and top with the pancakes.

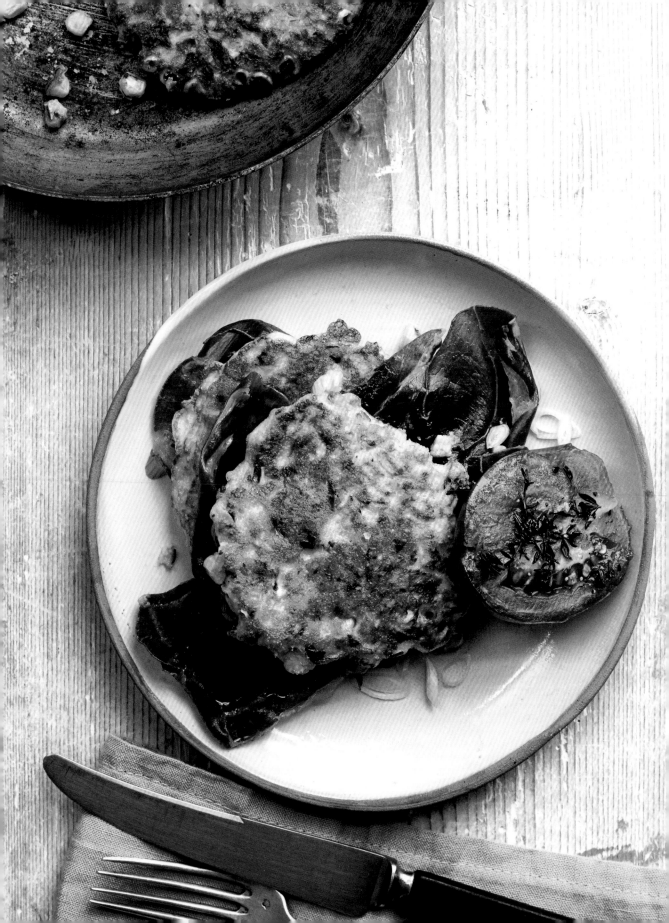

Spiced apricot & almond porridge

Porridge is a winning breakfast for when I'm training because its slow-releasing carbohydrates help me sustain my energy levels. I've given this recipe a little makeover and added fresh apricots for added vitamin A, which is great for immunity, and whole almonds, which have heaps of health-boosting nutrients. See my tips below for extra twists.

SERVES 2
324 calories per serving

70g oats

20g creamed coconut

1/2 tsp ground cinnamon, plus a pinch or two to serve (optional)

3 apricots, very finely chopped

8 whole almonds, finely chopped

2 tbsp coconut yoghurt

1 Put the oats into a medium saucepan and pour in 600ml water. Add the creamed coconut and cinnamon, if using. Place the pan over a medium heat and bring to the boil, stirring all the time. Lower the heat and cook for 3 minutes, allowing the mixture to bubble, until it starts to thicken.

2 Stir in the apricots and almost all of the almonds and cook for 1–2 minutes more so that the apricot starts to soften and cook into the porridge.

3 Spoon into two bowls, then top each bowl with a spoonful of yoghurt, the remaining almonds and a pinch or two of cinnamon, if liked.

TOM'S TIPS

Stir in a scoop of protein powder for an extra boost of protein.

For a treat, pop 1 square (5g) of dark chocolate (at least 70% cocoa solids) on top of the porridge to melt just before serving.

Raspberry & fig Bircher muesli

Bircher muesli is the original overnight oats recipe, created by a physician in the 1900s as a way to include more fresh fruit and vegetables into his patients' diets. Times haven't changed! I've added raspberries to this one with dried figs and flavoured it with cinnamon and lemon. Pear and apple work well – either in chunks or grated – but add them just before serving so they don't turn brown. Greek yoghurt is also packed with probiotics, which help to boost immunity.

SERVES 2
450 calories per serving

150g raspberries

2 dried figs, chopped

60g oats, lightly toasted in a dry frying pan

zest of 1/2 lemon

1 tsp ground cinnamon

150g Greek yoghurt

200ml milk

25g walnuts, finely chopped

1 This is really simple – just put everything into a bowl or container, stir together and cover with cling film or seal with a lid. Chill overnight.

2 When you're ready to eat breakfast, spoon into bowls and serve. I sometimes leave a few chopped walnuts to one side, so that I can sprinkle them over the top the next day for an extra crunch.

TOM'S TIPS

Add extra protein to this by stirring in a scoop of protein powder.

For a treat, grate one small square (around 5g) of dark chocolate (at least 70% cocoa solids) over the top.

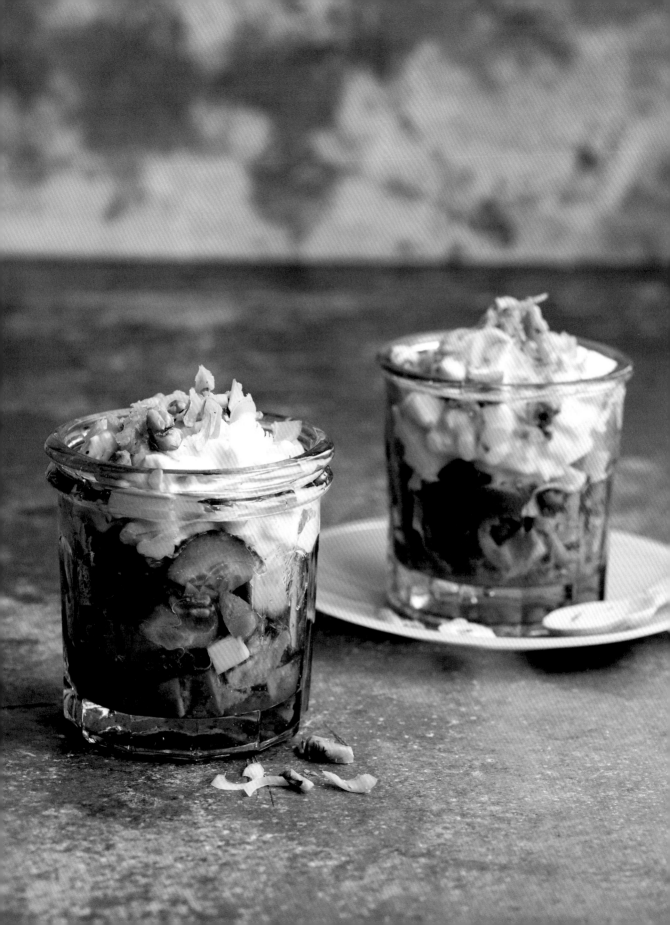

Cottage cheese pots

This is a bit of a twist on a yoghurt pot, with protein-packed cottage cheese as the main ingredient. Great for a summery breakfast, these pots can be prepared the night before and you're ready to go first thing! The base is finely chopped cucumber, tomato, avocado and spring onions, with black or green olives for extra flavour. Then it's topped with cottage cheese and walnuts.

SERVES 2
290 calories per serving

5cm chunk of cucumber, finely chopped

1 plum or vine tomato, finely chopped

1/2 avocado, finely chopped

2 spring onions, finely chopped

4 black or green stoned olives, chopped

1 tsp extra virgin olive oil

1/4 lemon

200g cottage cheese

6 walnuts, finely chopped

sea salt and freshly ground black pepper

1 Spoon the cucumber, tomato, avocado and half the chopped spring onions into a bowl. Add the olives and oil and squeeze over the lemon. Season well with salt and pepper and stir everything together.

2 Divide between two pots. Stir the remaining spring onions and the cottage cheese together and spoon on top of the mixed vegetables.

3 Sprinkle with the walnuts and top with a lid.

TOM'S TIP

For a sweet version, swap the vegetables for a mixture of summer fruits and add a squeeze of orange juice. Top with the cottage cheese and walnuts. I have had it in Eastern Europe and it's delicious!

light lunches & salads

Super-easy and full of flavour, these fresh lunch and salad recipes will keep your energy levels up, so say goodbye to late-afternoon snacking and energy dips.

Pea & ham soup

This recipe is a clever use of leftover ingredients from my one-pot gammon recipe in the Weekend Feasts chapter (see page 150). There's no need to season it as the stock is quite salty – just add plenty of black pepper at the end.

SERVES 2
330 calories per serving

700ml gammon stock (see page 150)

2 chunks of leftover cooked leek (see page 150)

4 leftover cooked potato halves, roughly chopped (see page 150)

150g frozen peas (no need to defrost)

150g leftover cooked gammon

freshly ground black pepper

1 Pour the stock into a saucepan and add the leek, potatoes and peas. Cover the pan with a lid and bring to the boil.

2 Reduce the heat a little and simmer for 5 minutes. Remove from the heat and use a hand-held blender to blitz the soup until smooth.

3 Shred the cooked gammon and stir into the soup; continue to simmer until the ham has warmed through. Ladle into bowls, season with black pepper and serve.

TOM'S TIP
You can easily double up this recipe. To freeze extra portions, just pour them into a sealable container, cool and transfer to the freezer. Label the box and use within 3 months.

Thai-style squash & noodle soup

I love a one-pot recipe as there's less washing-up to do and they're often quicker to rustle up, too. Feel free to switch up the veg, depending on what you have to hand – sweet potato would be a good alternative to the squash, for instance. Just check it's cooked before you add the noodles by pushing the point of a sharp knife into a piece.

SERVES 2
474 calories per serving

2 tsp coconut oil

1 red chilli

5cm piece of fresh root ginger, peeled and chopped into matchsticks

2 shallots, sliced

400g squash, peeled and chopped into 1–2cm cubes

1 litre hot light vegetable stock

100g rice noodles

100g sugar snap peas, halved

1 large pak choi, chopped

120g firm tofu, chopped into 1–2cm cubes

10g peanuts, toasted

small handful of basil leaves, to serve

1 Put the coconut oil, chilli, ginger and shallots into a large pan or wok and place over a medium heat. Cook for 3–4 minutes, stirring regularly, until the shallots start to turn golden and the chilli softens.

2 Add the squash and continue to cook for 3–4 minutes, again until the cubes start to turn golden and caramelise.

3 Pour in 600ml of the hot stock and simmer for 5 minutes. Add the noodles to the pan then pour the remaining stock over the top to cover them, dunking them under the liquid if you need to, to help them soften. Simmer for 3 minutes, or until just tender.

4 Add the sugar snap peas, pak choi and tofu and simmer again for another minute until the vegetables are tender and the tofu is warm.

5 Take the pan off the heat. Scatter the peanuts and basil leaves on top and serve.

TOM'S TIP
For a packed lunch, divide the oil, chilli, ginger, shallots, noodles, sugar snap peas and pak choi between two containers. Add ½ finely sliced pepper, the tofu, peanuts and 2 tsp powdered stock. To serve, pour in 450ml boiling water. Stir and wait 5 minutes until tender.

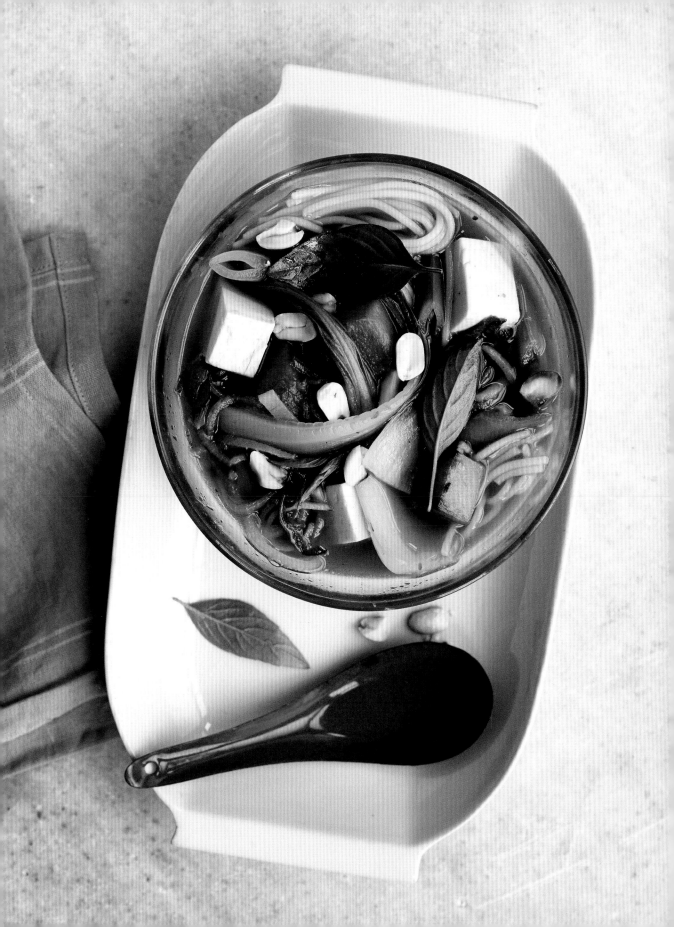

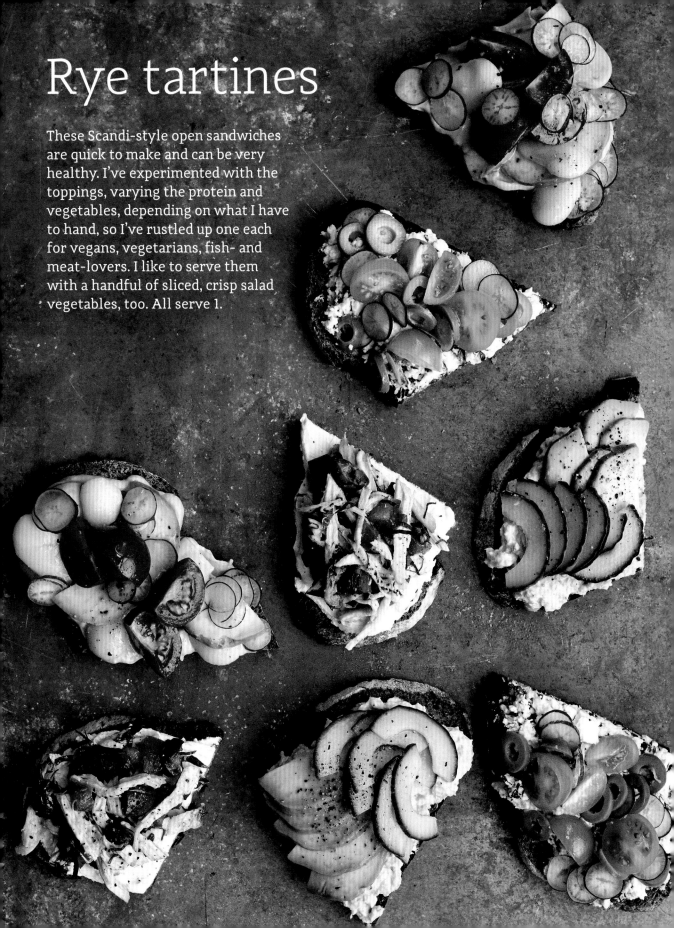

Rye tartines

These Scandi-style open sandwiches are quick to make and can be very healthy. I've experimented with the toppings, varying the protein and vegetables, depending on what I have to hand, so I've rustled up one each for vegans, vegetarians, fish- and meat-lovers. I like to serve them with a handful of sliced, crisp salad vegetables, too. All serve 1.

Tartine for vegans

264 calories per serving

1 slice of dark rye and sunflower bread
1 tbsp hummus
50g butterbeans
4 cherry tomatoes, quartered
2 radishes, thinly sliced
¼ small avocado, chopped
½ tsp extra virgin olive oil
freshly ground black pepper

1 Put the rye bread on a plate and spread the hummus over the top. Mix the butterbeans, cherry tomatoes, radishes, avocado and oil in a small bowl then spoon on top of the hummus.

2 Season with black pepper and serve.

Tartine for vegetarians

300 calories per serving

1 slice of dark rye and sunflower bread
50g feta cheese
1 tbsp Greek yoghurt
1 tbsp chopped parsley
1 tsp extra virgin olive oil
2 radishes, thinly sliced
4 cherry tomatoes, halved
4 olives, thinly sliced
freshly ground black pepper

1 Put the rye bread on a board. Mash the feta, yoghurt, parsley and olive oil in a bowl and spoon on top of the rye bread, spreading it out to the edges.

2 Scatter over the radishes, cherry tomatoes and olives then season and serve.

Tartine for fish-lovers

303 calories per serving

1 slice of dark rye and sunflower bread
1 tbsp Greek yoghurt
105g can pink salmon, drained
2cm piece of cucumber, chopped
¼ avocado, chopped
freshly ground black pepper

1 Put the rye bread on a plate. Put the yoghurt and salmon into a bowl and mash together. Spread over the rye bread then top with the cucumber and avocado.

2 Season with pepper and serve.

Tartine for meat-lovers

237 calories per serving

1 slice of dark rye and sunflower bread
1 tbsp light or reduced-fat cream cheese
1 medium vine tomato, chopped
3 black or green olives, stoned and finely chopped
1 tbsp chopped parsley
50g roast chicken, ham or roast beef, shredded
½ tsp extra virgin olive oil
freshly ground black pepper

1 Put the rye bread on a plate. Spread the cream cheese over the rye bread. Mix together the tomato, olives, parsley, cooked meat and oil and season with pepper.

2 Spoon on top of the cheese and serve.

Warm salmon salad

This protein-packed salad calls for a can of salmon, which is full of those essential omega-3s we all need (great for skin and joints). It makes a brilliant take-to-work lunch, too.

SERVES 2
390 calories per serving

TOM'S TIP

You can make this salad the night before. I mix the dressing into the salmon, then layer the other vegetables on top, which stops them becoming soggy.

150g green beans, halved

½ each red and yellow pepper, deseeded and thinly sliced

¼ red onion, thinly sliced

200g can kidney beans, drained

2 tbsp extra virgin olive oil

juice of ¼ lemon

15g parsley, finely chopped

6 stoned olives, finely chopped

213g can wild Pacific pink salmon, flaked into pieces

sea salt and freshly ground black pepper

1 Put the green beans, sliced peppers and onion into a saucepan and pour over enough water to just cover the vegetables. Put a lid on the pan, bring to the boil and simmer for 2–3 minutes until the vegetables are just tender.

2 Drain well and return to the pan. Stir in the kidney beans, olive oil, lemon juice, parsley and olives. Divide between two plates and top with the flaked salmon. Season with salt and pepper.

Autumn salad

Chunks of squash become the hero vegetable in this warm vegan salad, dotted with protein-rich butterbeans and topped with a non-creamy dressing made with tahini. I guarantee no one will miss the meat, as the flavours are so rich.

SERVES 2
460 calories per serving

large chunk of squash (about 325g)

1 red onion, cut into 6 wedges

1 small fennel bulb, cut into 4–6 wedges

2 tbsp extra virgin olive oil

10g whole almonds, finely chopped

10g pistachios, finely chopped

1/2 x 400g can butterbeans, drained (see Tom's Tip to use the other half of the can)

1 pear, thinly sliced

juice of 1/2 lemon

2 tbsp tahini

10g parsley, chopped

sea salt and freshly ground black pepper

1 Preheat the oven to its highest setting, usually 240°C/220°C Fan/Gas 9.

2 Put the squash, onion and fennel into a large bowl and pour over 1 tablespoon of the oil and 1 tablespoon of water. Season well and toss everything together. Tip into a roasting tin (set the bowl aside – you're going to use it for the next bit) and roast the vegetables in the oven for 20–25 minutes until soft, golden, tender and caramelised.

3 Meanwhile, put the remaining tablespoon of oil into the large bowl with the almonds, pistachios, butterbeans and sliced pear. Season and toss everything together.

4 When the vegetables are ready, spoon the butterbean mixture over the roasted vegetables and return to the oven for 5 minutes to warm through.

5 Mix the lemon juice, tahini and 2 tablespoons of water together in a bowl to make a dressing. Drizzle over the vegetables then scatter over the parsley and serve.

TOM'S TIP
Save the leftover butterbeans for Rye tartines (see page 99).

Crayfish cocktail with a Mexican twist

I've given the 70s' classic prawn cocktail a makeover with this salad, using little gem instead of iceberg lettuce, which provides the perfect cup shape to hold the filling. It's super-quick to make and super-tasty, too.

SERVES 2
152 calories per serving

¼ small red onion, finely chopped

juice of ½ lime

¼ green pepper, finely chopped

75g cherry tomatoes, chopped

½ medium avocado, chopped

finely sliced red chilli (optional)

1 tsp olive oil

120g crayfish tails

small handful of chopped coriander

1 little gem lettuce, leaves separated

sea salt and freshly ground black pepper

1 Put the onion into a bowl and pour the lime juice over the top. Season well with salt and pepper and stir together.

2 Add the pepper, cherry tomatoes, avocado, red chilli, if using, olive oil and crayfish tails and stir again, then gently fold in the coriander, reserving a little for garnish, if you like.

3 Spread the lettuce leaves over a plate then spoon the chopped salad all over the lettuce cups, scattering any reserved coriander on top. Serve at once.

TOM'S TIP
Prawns make a very easy alternative to the crayfish.

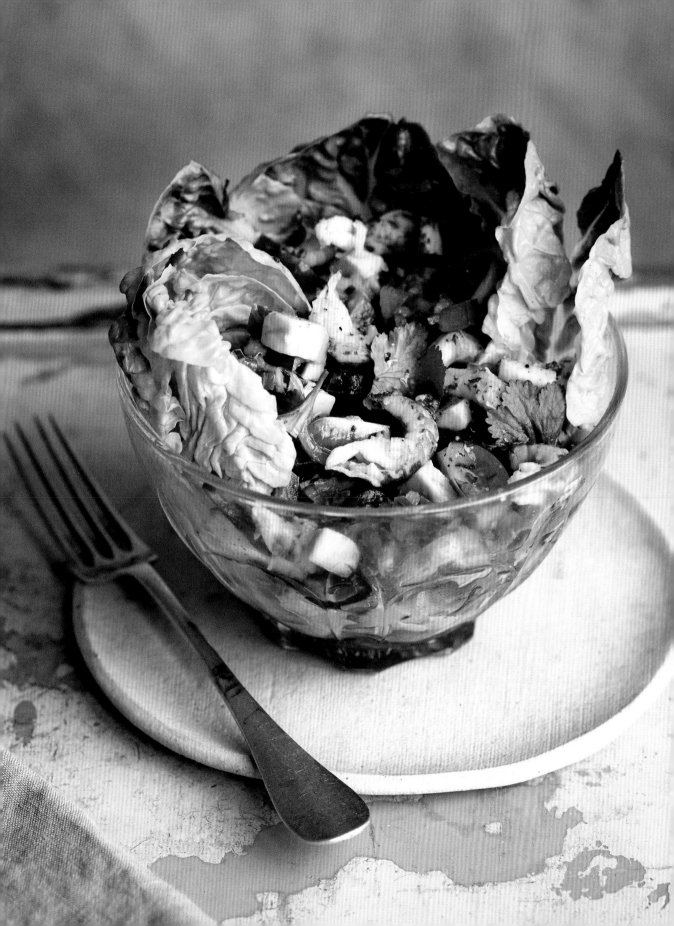

Italian salad

Mozzarella is at the heart of this salad, which mixes grilled veg – a great short cut to roasting – with crunchy giant croutons and a punchy rocket dressing. For an occasional treat, I swap the mozzarella for burrata. It looks like mozzarella on the outside (because it is!) and is more like curd or fresh cream on the inside.

SERVES 2
561 calories per serving

2 small courgettes

2 plum tomatoes, halved

1 garlic clove, halved

100g sourdough roll, cut into chunky croutons

60g bag of rocket

2 tbsp olive oil, plus extra for brushing

10g whole almonds

2 tsp red wine vinegar

1/2 x 400g can borlotti beans, drained (see tip below)

125g ball mozzarella, halved

sea salt and freshly ground black pepper

1 Preheat the grill.

2 Cut the courgettes in half lengthways, then each half in half to make two shorter pieces. Put on a baking sheet with the halved plum tomatoes.

3 Rub the halved garlic clove all over the cut side of the courgettes and tomatoes, then over the croutons. Brush the vegetables and croutons with oil and then pop the vegetables under the grill for 15 minutes. Add the croutons to the tray and grill for a few minutes more until golden, turning regularly.

4 Put half the rocket into a mini processor with the 2 tablespoons of oil, the almonds, red wine vinegar and 1 tablespoon of water. Season well then blitz until smooth. Mix 1 tablespoon of this dressing with the beans then divide the beans between two plates. Top with the courgettes, tomatoes and croutons and tear over the mozzarella. Add the remaining rocket then drizzle 1/2 tablespoon of dressing over each plate and serve.

TOM'S TIP
Spoon the remaining half can of borlotti beans into a small container and top with the remaining dressing. Store in the fridge and use in my Buddha bowl recipe on page 110.

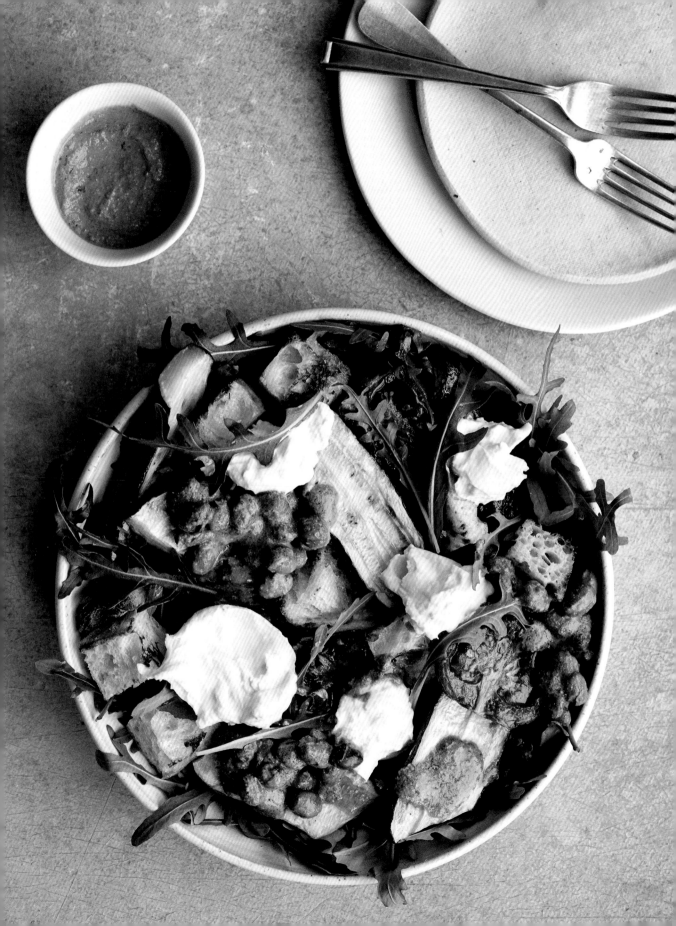

Mediterranean mezze salad

This deli-style supper brings some of my favourite ingredients together with a couple of healthy ready-made offerings. It combines hummus lightened with yoghurt, a quick one-pan chickpea dish, stuffed vine leaves and salad. It's great for a quick weekend lunch and the chickpeas can be made ahead and tumbled into a lunchbox to take to work.

SERVES 2
485 calories per serving

100g ready-made hummus

2 tbsp Greek yoghurt

1 tbsp extra virgin olive oil

2 spring onions, chopped

75g cherry tomatoes, quartered

400g can chickpeas, drained

1 tsp ground coriander

½ tsp paprika

sea salt and freshly ground black pepper

To serve

1 wholemeal pitta bread

4 stuffed vine leaves

5cm piece of cucumber, cut into batons

1 small lettuce such as little gem or chicory, sliced into wedges

1 Stir the hummus and Greek yoghurt together and pile into the centre of a large platter.

2 Heat ½ tablespoon of the olive oil in a saucepan and add the spring onions, tomatoes, chickpeas and spices and season well with salt and pepper. Add 5 tablespoons of water – this helps to cook the spices and also makes a little bit of a sauce – and simmer for 5 minutes to cook everything, stirring every now and then.

3 Toast the pitta bread while the chickpeas are cooking, then slice into fingers on a board.

4 Arrange the stuffed vine leaves, cucumber batons, lettuce and pitta around the hummus, then top with the spicy chickpeas and serve.

Warm quinoa salad with kale crisps

Quinoa is a powerhouse of nutrition as it contains all the essential amino acids and is a good source of protein – great if you're trying to include more non-meat options in your diet. Here it's steamed with vegetables, cooked until just tender and topped with kale crisps. Use feta in place of tofu if you eat dairy.

SERVES 2
400 calories per serving

100g quinoa

400ml hot vegetable stock

150g frozen peas (no need to defrost)

1 large carrot, diced, grated or shredded

2 spring onions, roughly chopped

1 tbsp extra virgin olive oil

juice of 1/2 lemon

10g soft herbs, such as parsley, chives or coriander, roughly chopped

100g firm tofu or feta cheese, diced

For the kale crisps

100g cavolo nero or kale, tough stems removed and leaves finely chopped

1 Put the quinoa into a saucepan and pour over about 300ml of the stock. Cover the pan with a lid and bring to the boil. Turn the heat down low and simmer for 10–12 minutes.

2 Stir in the peas, carrot and spring onions and cover with a lid again. Continue to cook over a low heat for 5 more minutes until the vegetables have steamed through and the quinoa is cooked.

3 Meanwhile, make the kale crisps. Preheat the grill and put the chopped kale in a bowl. Stir in 1 teaspoon of the olive oil, spread out on a baking sheet and grill until golden. You need to watch it carefully – I find it always burns the minute I turn my back!

4 Stir the remaining oil and the lemon juice through the quinoa, along with the herbs. Divide between two bowls and top with the tofu or feta. Finally, add the kale crisps and serve.

TOM'S TIPS

Season the kale with whatever spices you have to hand – chilli powder and smoked paprika work well.

No time to make the crisps? Just stir the kale into the quinoa along with the other vegetables.

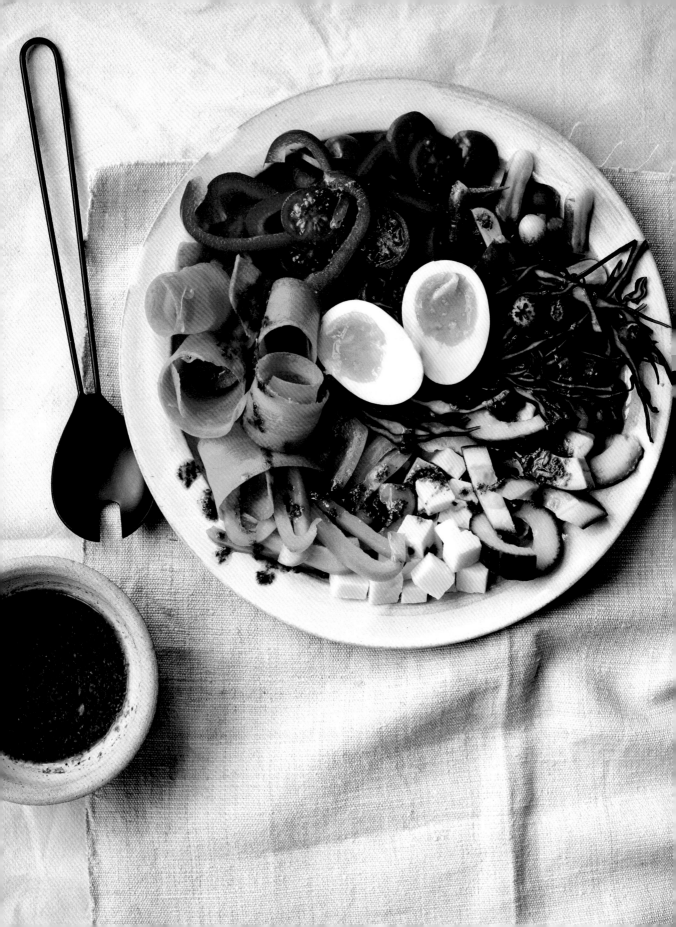

Tom's rainbow salad

I love combining fruit with crisp, raw vegetables, so have brought in blueberries to complete my rainbow salad. It's topped with boiled eggs and fingers of cheese but you could also use shredded chicken if you prefer meat, or chunks of tofu to make it vegan.

SERVES 2
445 calories per serving

For the salad

2 large eggs, at room temperature

½ medium red pepper, thinly sliced or 1 head of red chicory, shredded

8–10 cherry tomatoes, halved

½ medium yellow pepper, thinly sliced

6–8 radishes, halved

¼ cucumber, cut into batons

½ avocado, sliced

1 medium carrot, shredded

small chunk of red cabbage (about 100g), shredded

100g blueberries

50g light or reduced-fat Cheddar cheese, cut into thick cubes or fingers

For the dressing

1 sprig of basil

2 tbsp extra virgin olive oil

1 tbsp red wine vinegar

sea salt and freshly ground black pepper

1 Bring a small saucepan of water to the boil. Carefully lower the eggs into the pan, turn down the heat a little and simmer for 6 minutes. Spoon into a bowl of cold water and set aside.

2 Arrange the red pepper, cherry tomatoes, yellow pepper, radishes, cucumber, avocado, carrot, red cabbage and blueberries around the edge of a large platter.

3 Make the dressing. Put the leaves from the basil sprig into a mini processor or blender with the olive oil, vinegar and ½ tablespoon of boiling water. Season well and blitz until smooth.

4 Lift the eggs out of the cold water and crack on a board. Carefully peel the eggs then slice in half and place in the middle of the salad, along with the cheese.

5 Drizzle the dressing over the top, season and serve.

Tom's Buddha bowl

I try to eat vegan at least one day per week and this is a great way of making a meal out of leftovers from the fridge. I've used leftover borlotti beans and dressing here with some grilled broccoli, seeds and a very quick-to-make coleslaw. Borlotti beans are packed with potassium, which supports heart health, muscles and bone strength.

SERVES 2
367 calories per serving

For the bowl

150g tenderstem or purple sprouting broccoli, halved through the stem

olive or coconut oil

leftover borlotti beans and dressing (see Italian salad, page 104)

150g firm tofu, cut into cubes

1 tbsp mixed seeds (sunflower, pumpkin and sesame), toasted

For the coleslaw

1 small carrot, shredded

small chunk of red cabbage

1/2 red pepper, very thinly sliced

2 tbsp chopped fresh chives

juice of 1/4 lemon

sea salt and freshly ground black pepper

1 Preheat the grill. Brush the broccoli with the oil and grill until golden, turning halfway through.

2 Divide the borlotti beans and the dressing into two serving bowls and set aside.

3 Mix the carrot, cabbage, red pepper and chives for the coleslaw together with the lemon juice and season well. Divide between the two bowls, then top with the grilled broccoli, tofu and seeds. Serve at once.

I ALSO EAT THIS WITH REGULAR BROCCOLI AND CAULIFLOWER INSTEAD OF TENDERSTEM, COOKED IN THE SAME WAY – DELICIOUS!

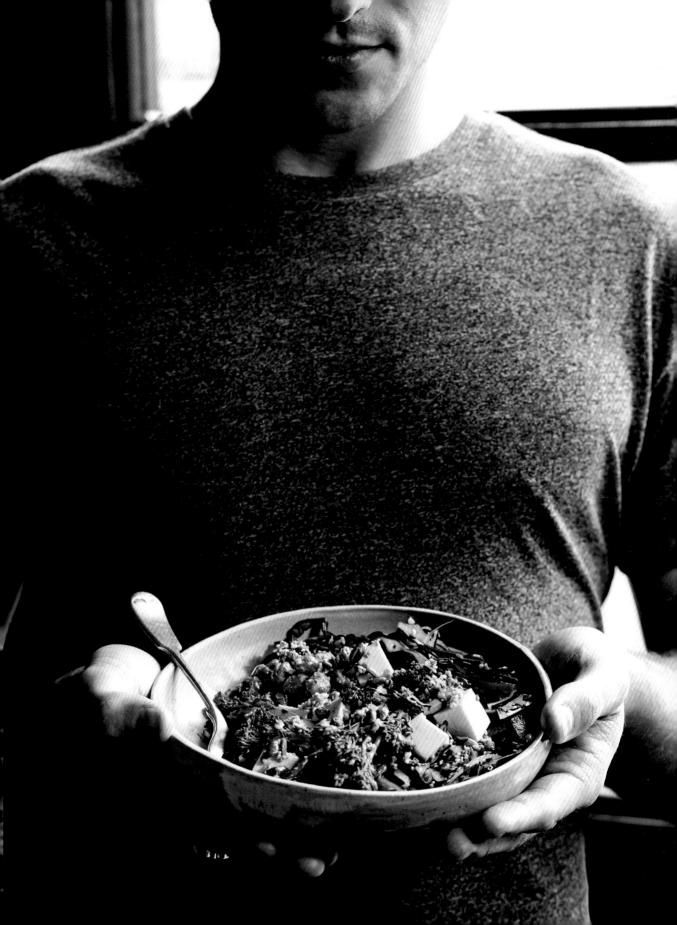

Chicken satay
with Asian slaw

Have you seen those little packets of uncut stir-fry vegetables in supermarkets, the ones with a couple of handfuls of different varieties, such as baby corn and tenderstem broccoli? I've used one in this recipe – they're convenient because they contain just the right amount of vegetables for this quick slaw. Pouring over the juices from the chicken at the end gives them extra flavour.

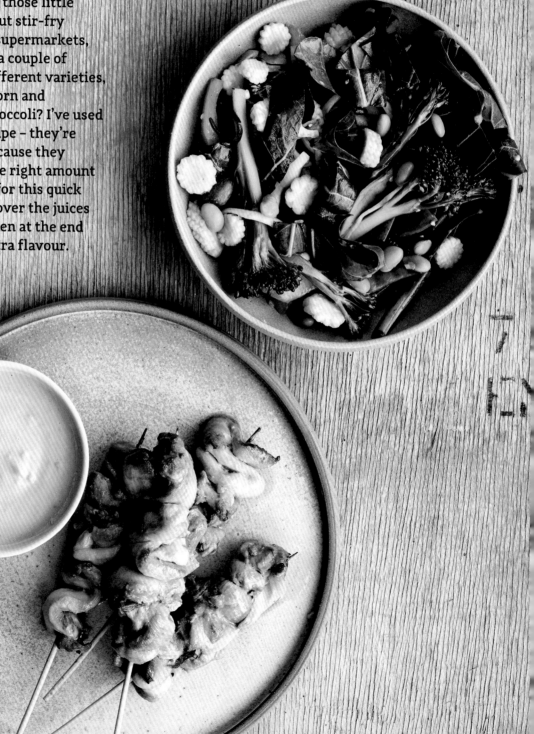

SERVES 2

470 calories per serving

1 packet of stir-fry vegetable medley, including baby corn, mangetout and tenderstem broccoli, shredded (set the chilli to one side)

1 tbsp soy sauce

1 tbsp sesame oil

juice of 1 lime

325g skinless and boneless chicken thighs, cut into finger-width strips

2 tbsp peanut butter

sea salt and freshly ground black pepper

1 Preheat the grill. Soak 6–8 wooden skewers in a bowl of warm water.

2 Put the shredded vegetables into a large bowl and stir in 1 teaspoon of the soy sauce, 1 teaspoon of the sesame oil and half the lime juice. Thinly slice half the chilli and add to the bowl then season well and stir everything together.

3 Put the chicken into a separate bowl and stir in 1 teaspoon of the soy sauce, 1 teaspoon of the sesame oil and half the remaining lime juice. Chop the remaining piece of chilli and add to the bowl. Season well and toss all the ingredients together.

4 Drain the skewers and then thread the chicken on to them. If you have short ones, you'll probably use eight skewers but if they're long, six will be enough. Lay the skewers on a baking tray and grill for 15 minutes, turning halfway through.

5 Meanwhile, make the satay sauce: put the peanut butter into a small bowl, add the remaining soy sauce, sesame oil and lime juice and 2 tablespoons of water. Stir well until smooth.

6 Check the chicken is cooked by cutting through one of the thickest parts on one of the skewers – it's ready when there is no visible pink meat and all the juices are clear.

7 Drizzle the juices over the shredded vegetables and stir in with a teaspoon of the satay sauce. Mix well and divide between two plates. Top with the chicken skewers and serve with the satay sauce.

ready in 15

In a hurry? My Ready-in-15 meals are ideal when you are short of time. These dishes can be whipped up in minutes and either eaten on the spot or taken to work.

Pea & tomato omelette with feta

Omelettes are the ultimate healthy fast food. I've made this one with frozen peas and tomatoes – both good sources of fibre – and added a little crumbled feta for flavour at the end.

SERVES 1
337 calories per serving

1 tsp coconut or olive oil

1 tomato, cut into 6–8 wedges

2 medium eggs

1 tbsp chopped parsley

75g frozen peas, defrosted

25g feta, crumbled

sea salt and freshly ground black pepper

1 Heat the oil in a large frying pan over a medium heat and add the tomato wedges. Cook on each side for 20–30 seconds until golden.

2 Beat the eggs in a bowl with most of the parsley and some salt and pepper. Pour into the frying pan and tilt the pan backwards and forward so it covers the base, then spoon the peas over the top.

3 With the pan still over a medium heat, use a spatula to pull the set edges of the egg into the middle to create holes, then tilt the pan again to let any uncooked egg run into the holes. Continue to do this until the egg has all cooked or set.

4 Scatter over the crumbled feta and remaining parsley, slide on to a plate and serve.

TOM'S TIP
To defrost peas in a hurry, put them in a small bowl and pour over enough boiling water to just cover. Leave for 1–2 minutes, then drain.

Hot chilli prawns with crisp salad

Prawns are a flash-in-the-pan fish as they cook so quickly – they're ready when they've turned from grey to pink. These are flavoured with spring onion and chilli for a bit of a kick and served on top of a bowlful of crisp vegetables.

SERVES 1
336 calories per serving

1 pak choi, shredded

4 radishes, sliced

5 cherry tomatoes, halved

50g mangetout or sugar snap peas, halved

75g edamame beans

1 tsp sesame or coconut oil

150g raw, peeled tiger prawns, peeled and deveined

1 spring onion, finely chopped

½ red chilli, sliced

1 tsp soy sauce

1 tsp honey

sea salt and freshly ground black pepper

lime wedge (optional)

1 Put the pak choi into a serving bowl. Add the radishes, cherry tomatoes, mangetout or sugar snaps and edamame beans.

2 Heat the oil in a wok or medium frying pan; when the oil is hot, add the prawns, spring onion and chilli. Season well and stir-fry for 1–2 minutes until the prawns have turned pink. Add the soy sauce, honey and 2 tablespoons of water and then take the pan immediately off the heat.

3 Toss to mix everything together then spoon the prawns and warm dressing over the salad vegetables. Serve with a lime wedge, if you like.

TOM'S TIP

Keep a bag of frozen edamame beans in the freezer for this. To defrost quickly, measure the required quantity into a bowl, cover with boiling water and leave for 2–3 minutes, then drain well.

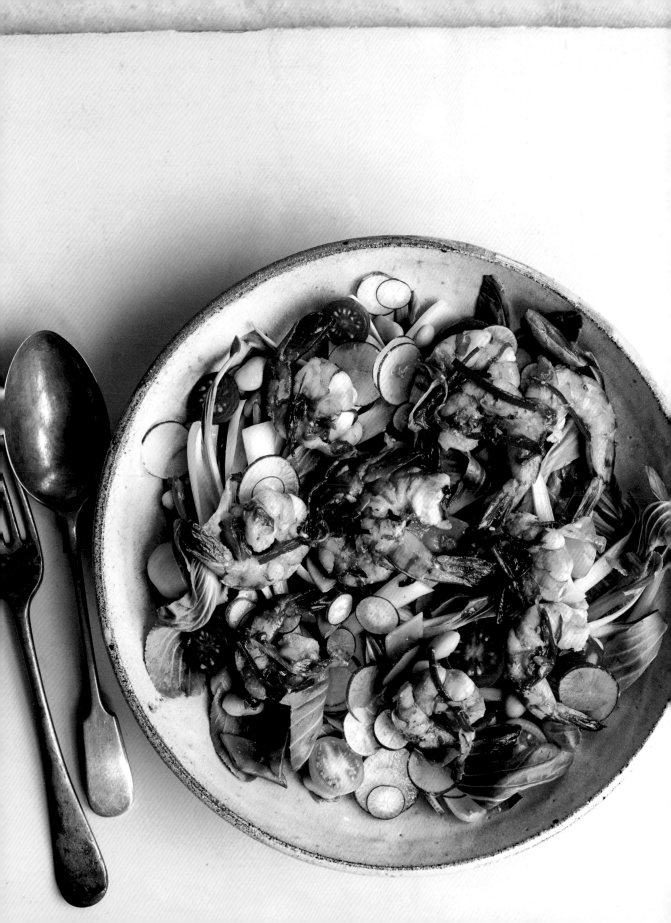

Quick healthy fried eggs

There's no need to use loads of oil when frying eggs, as this recipe shows. Just stir-fry some chopped vegetables first, then make a hole in the middle and drop in two eggs. Cover the pan and cook over a medium heat until the whites have set and the yolk is still runny.

SERVES 1
333 calories per serving

1 tsp coconut oil

1/2 red onion, chopped

1/2 red pepper, deseeded and chopped

1 courgette (about 150g), chopped

100g cherry tomatoes, halved

2 medium eggs

10g Parmesan cheese

sea salt and freshly ground black pepper

1 Heat the oil in a medium or large frying pan over a medium heat. Add the onion, pepper and courgette. Season well with salt and pepper and cook for 2–3 minutes, stirring.

2 Add the cherry tomatoes to the pan and continue to cook the vegetables for 4 minutes until golden and tender, tossing every now and then.

3 Push the vegetables aside with your wooden spoon to make two holes, then crack an egg into each one. Cover with a lid and cook for 2–3 minutes until the whites are set – a see-through lid is really handy, if you have one, to check on how the eggs are cooking.

4 Once the eggs are done the way you like them, grate over the Parmesan and serve.

MATURE CHEDDAR WORKS REALLY WELL IF I DON'T HAVE ANY PARMESAN IN THE FRIDGE

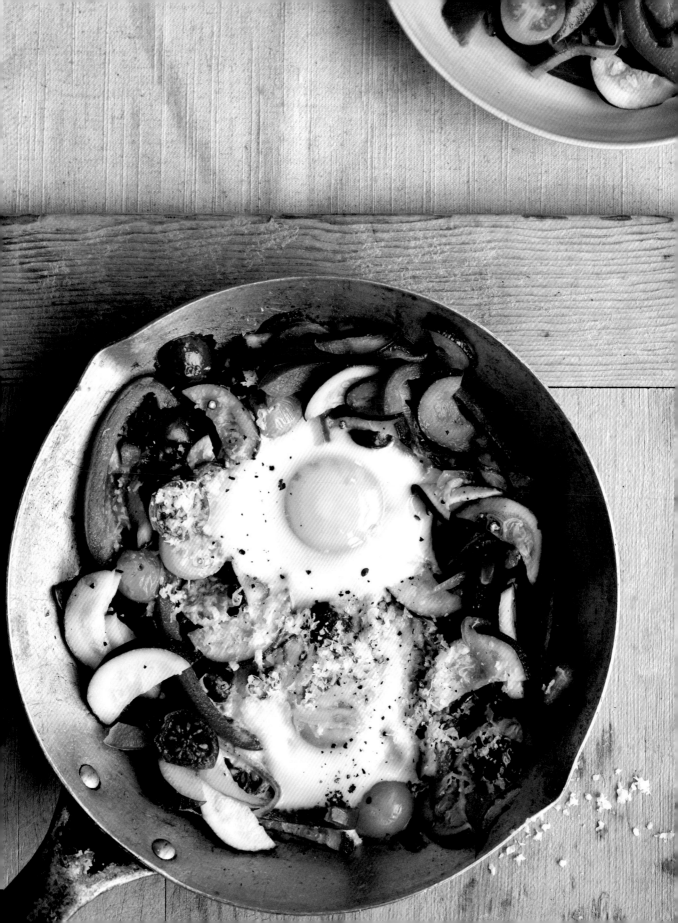

Quick lemon chicken with steamed veg

Squeezing lemon over chicken makes it deliciously tender, even if you do this just before cooking. If you want to get ahead, you could prepare the chicken in the morning and keep it chilled until the evening.

SERVES 1
302 calories per serving

125–150g skinless chicken breast or thigh fillet

juice of 1/2 lemon

2 tsp olive oil

250g mixed vegetables, such as green beans, asparagus, tenderstem broccoli, cauliflower florets and Chantenay carrots, halved or trimmed into even-sized pieces

sea salt and freshly ground black pepper

1 Cut the chicken into chunks, add to a bowl and pour over the lemon juice. Season with salt and pepper.

2 Heat the oil in a frying pan over a medium heat, then add the chicken and juice from the bowl. Spread the chicken pieces out slightly so that they brown nicely on one side, then turn over. Add 4 tablespoons of water to the pan, cover with a lid and cook for 10 minutes over a low heat until the chicken is cooked through.

3 Put the vegetables into a saucepan and pour in enough water to just cover them. Put a lid on the pan and steam over a high heat for 6–8 minutes. Drain well.

4 Arrange the vegetables on a plate then spoon the chicken on top and drizzle over the juices from the pan.

Speedy tofu pasta

Here's a super-quick pasta recipe using tofu. Chopping it really finely means it takes just minutes to cook. It does need seasoning though, so taste as you go and add more pepper or chilli flakes to get it how you like it.

SERVES 1
680 calories per serving

125g firm tofu

100g penne pasta

2 tsp olive oil

1 shallot, finely chopped

1 garlic clove, sliced

10g whole almonds, chopped

pinch of chilli flakes

zest of 1/2 lemon, plus the juice of 1/4 lemon

100g cavolo nero, chopped

10g parsley, finely chopped

sea salt and freshly ground black pepper

1 Boil a full kettle then pour the water into a medium saucepan and bring to the boil. Meanwhile, finely chop the tofu.

2 Add the pasta to the boiling water and cook for about 10 minutes, or until al dente.

3 Heat the oil in a frying pan over a medium heat and stir-fry the shallot, garlic, almonds and tofu for about 5 minutes until the shallot has softened.

4 Shake over the chilli flakes and season with salt and black pepper – taste a little to check the mixture is seasoned enough. Stir in the lemon zest.

5 About 3 minutes before the pasta has finished cooking, add the cavolo nero to the pan. Once the pasta is cooked, drain well and return to the pan. Add the tofu mixture, along with the lemon juice and parsley and stir everything together well. Taste again and season with more salt and pepper if it needs it. Spoon into a bowl and serve immediately.

IF I CAN'T FIND CAVOLO NERO IN MY LOCAL SHOPS, I SHRED SOME SAVOY CABBAGE INSTEAD

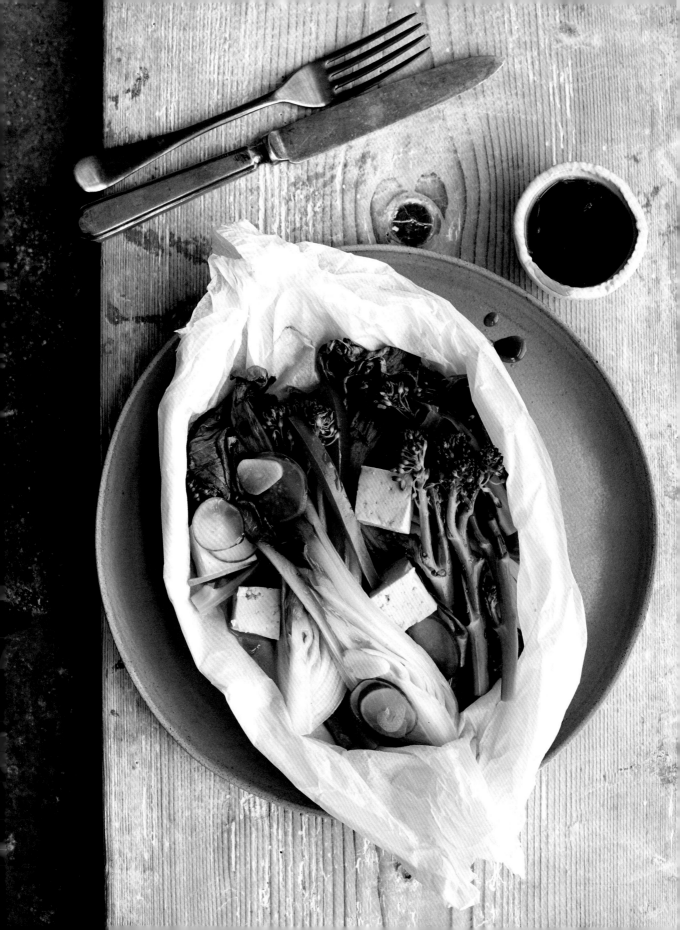

Steamed tofu parcel

This very simple recipe contains lots of crisp vegetables that need very little cooking so are ideal for a quick, post-workout dinner. Smoked tofu is great here as the flavour is delicious with the lime, maple syrup and soy sauce. It is also a great source of protein and all eight essential amino acids, which are important for muscle growth and repair.

SERVES 1
194 calories per serving

½ red pepper, deseeded and sliced

4 radishes, sliced

1 pak choi, quartered

4 tenderstem broccoli stems, thinly sliced

1 garlic clove, sliced

70g smoked tofu, cubed

juice of ½ lime

1 tsp maple syrup

2 tsp soy sauce

1 Cut a large square of baking parchment – don't use greaseproof paper or the parcel will fall apart. Spoon the pepper, radishes, pak choi, broccoli and garlic into the middle then place the smoked tofu on top. Bring the sides of the parchment together in the middle, fold over a couple of times, then twist the ends to wrap up into a parcel.

2 Pour boiling water into a saucepan to a depth of about 5cm, put a steamer or colander on top then place over a medium heat. Rest the parcel in the steamer or colander, cover with a lid and steam for 8–10 minutes, or until the vegetables are tender.

3 Whisk together the lime juice, maple syrup and soy sauce in a bowl with 1 teaspoon of boiling water.

4 Once the parcel is ready, lift out on to a plate and open it up. Pour over the dressing and serve.

TOM'S TIPS

This is so quick to prepare, but to save even more time at the end of your day you could get the parcel ready at breakfast time. Wrap it up and leave in the fridge until you're ready to cook.

No steamer? Use a colander or sieve resting over the pan.

Healthy steamed salmon

Here's another of my favourite one-pan dishes. The vegetables are lightly pan-fried first, then the salmon is tucked into the middle and cooked skin side down until crisp, then steamed until cooked through. The yoghurt and avocado mash, dolloped on at the end, isn't essential but it is an awesome addition.

SERVES 1
526 calories per serving

1 tsp olive oil

1 spring onion, roughly chopped

75g broccoli, cut into small florets

75g frozen peas, defrosted (see Tom's Tip on page 115)

good pinch of smoked or plain paprika

150g salmon fillet

1/4 avocado

1 tbsp Greek yoghurt

1 tbsp chopped chives or parsley (optional)

sea salt and freshly ground black pepper

lemon wedge, to serve

1 Heat the oil in a medium or large frying pan and stir-fry the onion, broccoli and peas with 1 tablespoon of water for a few minutes over a medium heat. Season with salt and pepper.

2 Sprinkle the paprika over the salmon and season with salt and pepper. Make a hole in the middle of the vegetables and place the salmon into the pan, skin side down. Cook for about 1 minute to crisp the skin, then add 2 more tablespoons of water to the pan and cover with a lid. Reduce the heat to low and steam for 4–5 minutes.

3 Meanwhile, mash the avocado with the yoghurt and the chives or parsley, if using.

4 Spoon the vegetables on to a plate and top with the salmon. Dollop with the avocado mash and serve with a lemon wedge.

TOM'S TIP
Oily fish, such as good-quality salmon or mackerel, is ideal after a workout as it's packed with anti-inflammatory omega-3 fats.

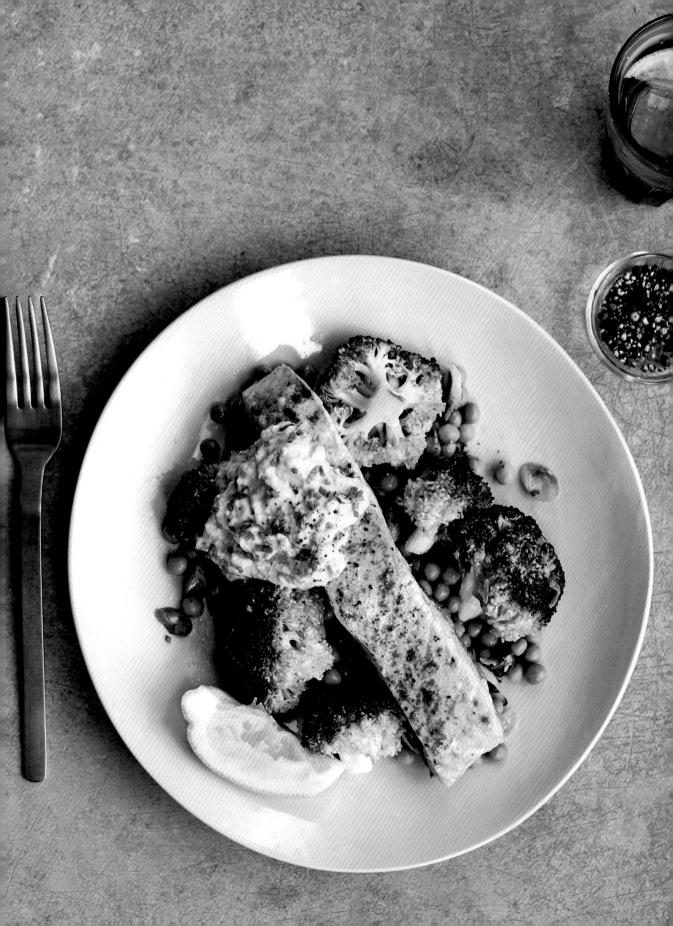

suppers

Feel inspired by my ideas for supper and dinners. From vegan baked peppers and teriyaki noodles, through to fishy feasts, there will be something here to satisfy everyone, whatever night of the week.

Tom's pesto pasta

Making your own pesto is a cinch with a mini processor – throw everything in and blitz – plus you can choose whatever you like to go into it. I've swapped pine nuts for brazil nuts and pumpkin seeds, which give it lots of flavour, plus I've added parsley, too.

SERVES 2
580 calories per serving

150g linguine

1 large courgette, spiralised or shredded with a serrated Y-peeler

150g frozen peas

2 spring onions, roughly chopped

For the pesto

4 brazil nuts

1 tbsp pumpkin seeds

2 sprigs of basil

small handful of parsley

2 tbsp olive oil

sea salt and freshly ground black pepper

1 Bring a large saucepan of water to the boil. As soon as the water is boiling, add the pasta, curling it round in the water and tucking it under the surface. Cook at a good simmer, following the timings on the packet.

2 While the pasta is cooking, make the pesto. Put the brazil nuts into a mini processor with the pumpkin seeds, basil, parsley and oil, along with a tablespoon of water. Season well and whizz until smooth.

3 Two minutes before the pasta is ready, drop the courgette strips, frozen peas and spring onions into the pan and continue to cook for the remaining time.

4 Drain the pasta and vegetables then return to the pan with a little bit of the cooking water still clinging to it. Add the pesto and stir in. Spoon between two bowls and serve.

TOM'S TIP
If you eat eggs, choosing fresh egg pasta will give you a small protein boost.

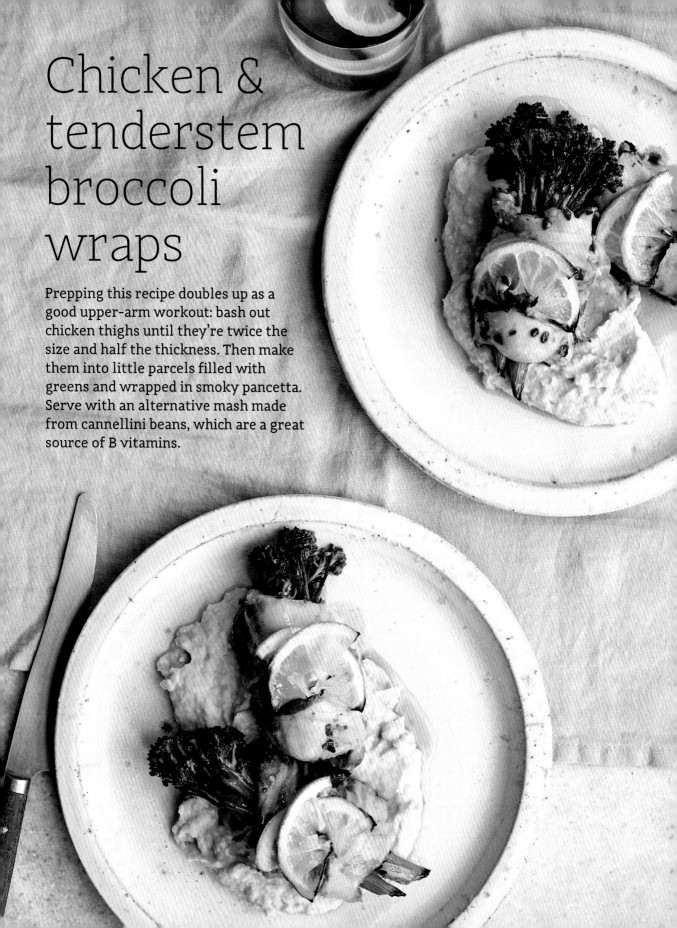

Chicken & tenderstem broccoli wraps

Prepping this recipe doubles up as a good upper-arm workout: bash out chicken thighs until they're twice the size and half the thickness. Then make them into little parcels filled with greens and wrapped in smoky pancetta. Serve with an alternative mash made from cannellini beans, which are a great source of B vitamins.

SERVES 2
550 calories per serving

200ml hot chicken or vegetable stock

8 stems of tenderstem or purple sprouting broccoli (about 200g)

4 skinless chicken thigh fillets

pinch of chilli flakes

2 tsp olive oil

4 slices of smoked pancetta

4 lemon slices

400g can cannellini beans, drained

sea salt and freshly ground black pepper

1 Preheat the oven to 200°C/180°C Fan/Gas 6.

2 Pour the stock into a medium saucepan and bring to a simmer. Add the broccoli, cover with a lid and cook for about 2 minutes, or until the stems turn bright green. They don't need to be cooked all the way through as they're going in the oven. Set aside to cool, reserving the stock in the pan.

3 Line a board with cling film then lay the chicken thighs on top, unrolling them so they're flat. Cover with another piece of cling film and bash with a rolling pin until they're more or less twice the size and half as thick.

4 Take the top layer of cling film off the chicken and scatter a good pinch of chilli flakes over each piece. Season well and drizzle each with 1/4 teaspoon of oil. Put two stems of broccoli in each flattened out piece of chicken and roll up, then wrap in a slice of pancetta. Place a lemon slice on top of each and secure the whole lot with a cocktail stick.

5 Put into a small roasting tin and drizzle each with another 1/4 teaspoon of oil. Drizzle in enough water to cover the base of the tin by about 5mm and transfer the tin to the oven to roast for 20 minutes.

6 Halfway through cooking the chicken, put the cannellini beans into the saucepan of reserved stock and season well. Bring to a simmer and cook over a low heat for 8 minutes, or until almost all of the stock has been absorbed. Mash well until smooth.

7 Divide the mash between two plates and top with the chicken and any juices in the roasting tin.

IF I FEEL LIKE RINGING THE CHANGES I USE PORK ESCALOPES INSTEAD. LEAN PORK IS A GREAT SOURCE OF PROTEIN

Baked peppers

These peppers are filled with a nourishing combination of protein-rich beans and nutritious sweet potatoes – a great GI vegetable that helps to control blood sugar – and baked until just tender. Serve with steamed greens.

SERVES 2
408 calories per serving

1 tbsp olive oil, plus a little extra for drizzling

1 shallot, finely chopped

1 small sweet potato or squash (about 150g), diced

1 tsp fajita spice mix

2 large peppers (any colour), halved and deseeded

25g wholemeal or sourdough bread, roughly chopped

1 tsp pumpkin seeds

400g can black-eyed beans, drained

sea salt and freshly ground black pepper

200g green beans, to serve

1 Preheat the oven to 200°C/180°C Fan/Gas 6.

2 Heat the oil in a frying pan. Add the shallot and sweet potato (or squash) and 1 tablespoon of water and cook over a low heat, stirring every now and then, for 5 minutes until softened and starting to turn golden. Stir in the fajita spice mix halfway through cooking and season well.

3 Meanwhile, put the peppers into a small roasting tin, cut side up. Put the bread chunks and pumpkin seeds into a mini processor and whizz to make breadcrumbs and to chop the seeds.

4 Add the drained beans to the frying pan and stir in, then spoon the mixture evenly into the halved peppers. Drizzle each pile of beans with a tablespoon of water. Scatter the breadcrumb mixture over the top and bake for 20 minutes until the peppers are tender.

5 While the peppers are cooking, steam the green beans until tender; they should take 4–5 minutes. Drain and return to the pan, then drizzle with about a teaspoon of oil and season well.

6 Transfer the peppers on to plates and serve with the steamed beans.

Parmesan cod with quick Mediterranean vegetables

Here's a one-pan supper that's ready in about half an hour. Don't cut the vegetables too small or they'll cook down into a mush – they should still be a little bit chunky when you come to tuck in. The stewed vegetables make the perfect base into which you nudge chunks of cod (or use any firm white fish you fancy).

SERVES 2
326 calories per serving

2 tbsp olive oil

1 small aubergine, cubed

1 red pepper, chopped

2 vine tomatoes, chopped

1 fat garlic clove, sliced

1 tbsp tomato purée

2 x 150g skinless cod fillets, cut into chunks

20g Parmesan cheese

small handful of soft herbs, such as parsley or chives, chopped

sea salt and freshly ground black pepper

1 Heat the oil in a large casserole, add the aubergine and peppers and cook over a low–medium heat for 7–8 minutes until the aubergine has softened and turned golden. Stir the vegetables every now and then to stop them sticking to the pan.

2 Stir in the vine tomatoes, garlic and tomato purée and cook for a further 2–3 minutes. Season well and then pour in 300ml water.

3 Bring to a simmer and cook for about 8 minutes, or until the base looks saucy. Add the cod chunks, tucking them slightly into the sauce. Cover the pan with a lid and cook over a low heat for 5 minutes until the fish is just opaque all the way through.

4 Just before serving, grate over the Parmesan and sprinkle with the herbs.

Tuna with mango & lime

Fresh tuna is a great source of omega-3s, the fatty acids important for heart and bone health, among other things. You can sear the steaks for as little or as long as you want to – the texture becomes meatier the longer it's in the pan. The vegetables I've chosen to go with this don't need cooking so they provide a lovely, crisp texture against the noodles and fish. All you do is stir them into the noodles to warm through in the heat of the pan.

SERVES 2
500 calories per serving

100g rice noodles

300g fresh tuna steak (about 1 thick slice)

2 pak choi, thinly sliced

1 corn on the cob, kernels sliced off (about 125g)

2 spring onions, sliced

1 red chilli, thinly sliced

zest of 1 lime

1 tsp toasted sesame seeds, to serve

For the dressing

½ large mango, diced

2 tsp toasted sesame oil, plus extra for drizzling

juice of 1 lime

sea salt and freshly ground black pepper

1 First, make the dressing. Put half the diced mango into a small blender or mini processor. Add the sesame oil and the lime juice. Season well and blitz until smooth.

2 Bring a large saucepan of water to the boil. Add the rice noodles to the pan then turn off the heat, give the noodles a stir and leave to soak for about 5 minutes, or according to the timings on the packet.

3 Drizzle a little oil over the tuna and rub in, then season well. Heat a non-stick frying pan until hot, add the tuna and cook over a medium heat for about 2 minutes each side – the tuna should still be pink in the middle.

4 Drain the noodles and return to the pan. Add the pak choi, sweetcorn, spring onions, chilli and half the lime zest. Stir everything together in the heat of the pan, then add the dressing and stir again.

5 Slice the tuna on a board into finger-width strips. Divide the noodle salad between two bowls, top with the tuna and the sesame seeds and scatter over a little extra lime zest.

TOM'S TIP

If you can't get fresh sweetcorn for this, use a drained 198g can, without sugar or salt.

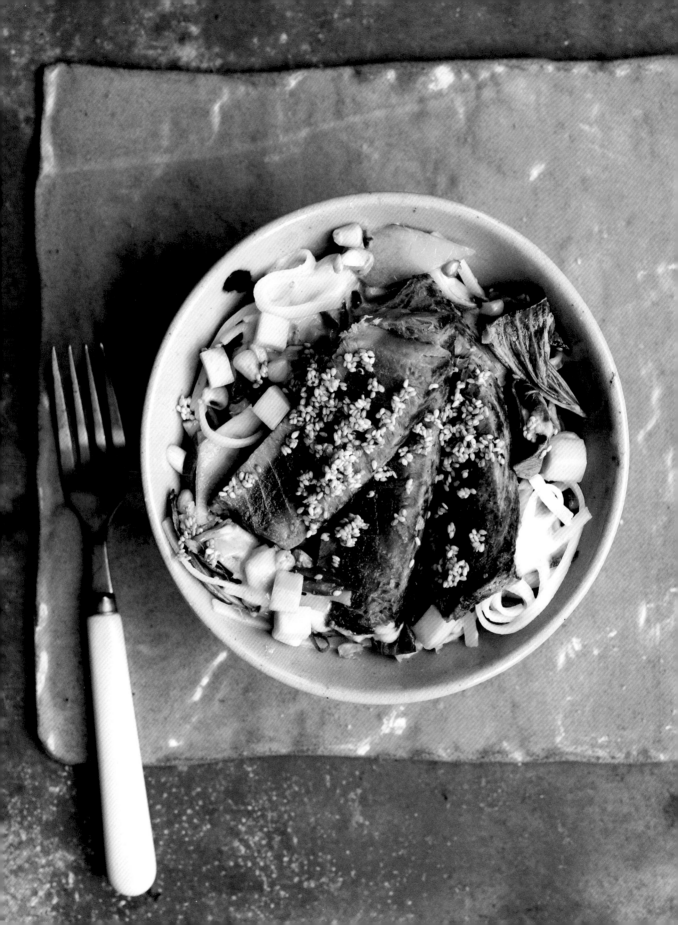

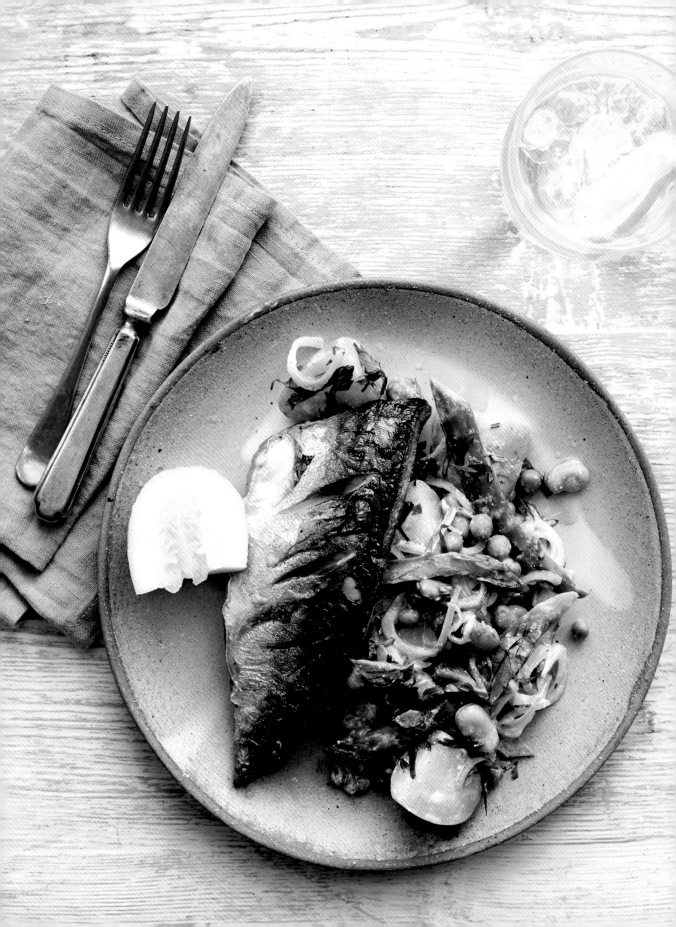

Pan-fried mackerel with new potato salad

Fillets of oily mackerel have lots of health benefits, including being rich in those essential omega-3 fatty acids and vitamin K, which boosts heart health. Serve with this simple chopped potato salad, packed with fibre-rich vegetables and tossed in a simple yoghurt dressing.

SERVES 2
606 calories per serving

1 shallot, thinly sliced

1 tsp white wine vinegar

200g new potatoes, quartered

100g fresh or frozen peas

100g asparagus

100g podded broad beans

1 tsp olive oil

2 x 150g mackerel fillets

2 tbsp Greek yoghurt

2 tbsp chopped parsley

1/2 lemon, cut into wedges

sea salt and freshly ground black pepper

1 Put the shallot into a small bowl. Add the vinegar and a pinch of salt and set aside.

2 Bring a medium saucepan of water to the boil. Add the potatoes and cook for 10 minutes, or until almost tender. Add the peas, asparagus and broad beans and continue to cook for a further 3 minutes until the potatoes and vegetables are tender.

3 Rub the oil all over the mackerel and season well with salt and pepper. Heat a griddle pan or frying pan until hot and fry the mackerel skin side down over a medium heat for 1–2 minutes, or until crisp. Flip over and cook for 1–2 minutes on the other side until the mackerel is cooked through.

4 When the potatoes and vegetables are cooked, drain well and return to the warm pan. Tip the shallot and vinegar into the pan, then add the Greek yoghurt and parsley. Season and mix everything together then divide between two plates.

5 Top with the mackerel and serve with the lemon wedges.

Salmon poké bowl

Have you heard of Hawaiian poké bowls? Lance and I went to Hawaii for our honeymoon and this was one of our favourite local dishes. They contain all the same elements as sushi, just not wrapped up! The base is usually sushi rice (or short-grain rice), topped with marinated raw fish and lots of fresh vegetables. If you don't fancy eating raw fish, lightly steam it first then toss in the dressing.

SERVES 2
714 calories per serving

100g short-grain brown rice

300g piece of very fresh salmon, cut into 2cm cubes

1 tsp soy sauce

1 tsp sesame oil

1 tsp grated ginger

10cm piece of cucumber, thinly sliced

2 spring onions, thinly sliced

1 tbsp white wine vinegar

pinch each of sugar and salt

160g frozen edamame beans, defrosted (see Tom's Tip on page 115)

½ small avocado, sliced

½ red chilli, sliced (optional)

1 tsp sesame seeds

½ lime, cut into wedges

1 Put the rice into a small saucepan and cover with plenty of boiling water. Cover the pan with a lid and bring to the boil. Turn the heat down to the lowest setting and cook at a very low simmer for 20–25 minutes, or until the rice is tender.

2 Put the salmon, soy sauce, sesame oil and ginger into a bowl and stir everything together. Set aside.

3 Put the cucumber and spring onions into a separate bowl and add the vinegar, sugar and salt. Stir and set aside.

4 When the rice is cooked, drain well. Drain the cucumber mixture. Divide the rice between two bowls, spreading it out over the base, then add the cucumber mixture, spooning it on top of one section of the rice. Add half the edamame beans to each bowl and half the avocado to cover the rice.

5 Finally spoon the salmon into the middle, along with the marinade. Scatter over the sliced chilli, if using, and sesame seeds. Serve with the lime wedges.

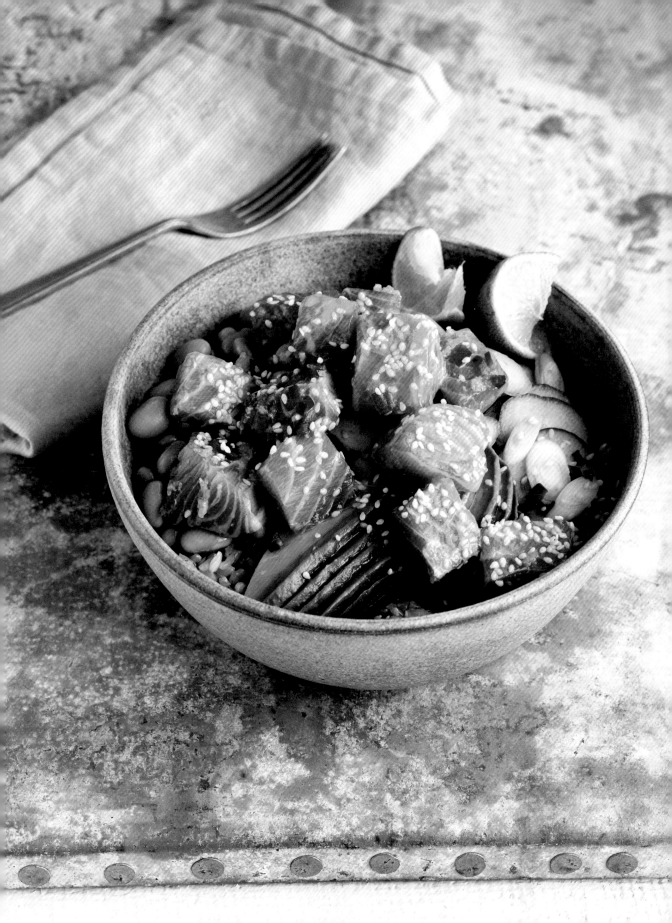

Sweet potato pan-fry with cheesy steak

Here's a great Friday night supper, so if you're feeling the urge to reach for the takeaway menu, make this instead – it'll be ready in half an hour! The pan-fry is just like a stir-fry, with slightly chunkier vegetables, tossed with a little balsamic vinegar at the end.

SERVES 2
433 calories per serving

1 tbsp olive oil, plus a little extra for frying the steak

1 sweet potato (about 160g), cut into 2cm cubes

1 red onion, roughly chopped

1 red pepper, deseeded and chopped

150g mixed green vegetables, such as broccoli and kale

250g rump steak

1–2 tsp balsamic vinegar

1 tbsp chopped parsley (optional)

10g Parmesan cheese

sea salt and freshly ground black pepper

lemon wedges, to serve (optional)

1 Heat 2 teaspoons of the oil in a large frying pan or wok and stir-fry the sweet potato for 5 minutes. Add the red onion and cook for a further 5 minutes, stirring every now and then.

2 Add the red pepper and greens to the pan and continue to cook for 5–7 minutes, tossing the vegetables regularly. Add 100ml water to the pan, season well, then turn the heat down to low and cover with a lid. Cook for 5 minutes.

3 Rub about ¼ teaspoon of oil all over the steak and season well with salt and pepper. Heat a small frying pan until hot and cook the steak for 2–3 minutes on each side, depending on the thickness.

4 Meanwhile, add the balsamic vinegar and remaining oil to the vegetables and stir in the parsley, if using.

5 Slice the steak on a board into finger-width strips. Divide the vegetables between two plates, top with the steak and grate the Parmesan over the top. Serve with a wedge of lemon to squeeze over the top, if liked.

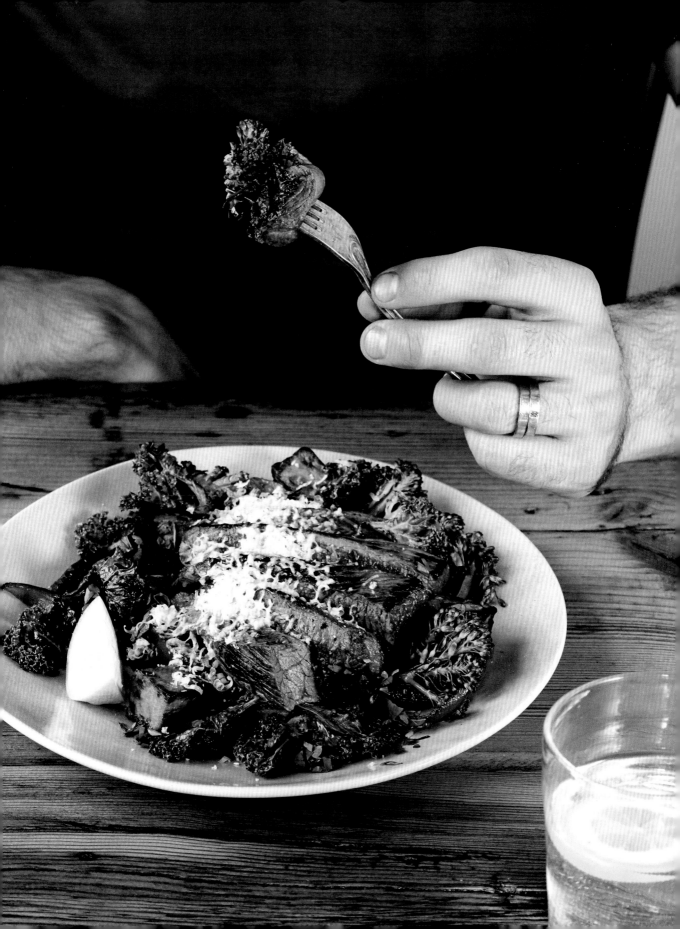

Chicken meatballs with orzo, parsley & lemon

These simple chicken meatballs, containing chopped dried apricots and topped with parsley and lemon, taste really special. It's worth making a batch to freeze, too. If you don't fancy serving these with the pasta and sauce, they are also delicious stuffed into a wholemeal pitta, with a drizzle of Greek yoghurt and lots of chopped salad.

SERVES 2
592 calories per serving

For the meatballs

about 300g skinless chicken breast fillet (or use turkey), roughly chopped

1 shallot, roughly chopped

4 apricots, chopped

2 tbsp oats

1 medium egg

1 tsp olive oil

sea salt and freshly ground black pepper

For the tomato sauce

1 tsp olive oil

2 garlic cloves, sliced

400g can chopped tomatoes

700ml hot chicken or vegetable stock

75g orzo pasta

100g frozen peas

zest 1/4 lemon

2 tbsp chopped parsley

1 Put the chicken into the bowl of a food processor and add the shallot, apricots, oats and egg. Season well and whizz everything together until the mixture is minced finely. Use a teaspoon to scoop out pieces of the mixture and roll in your hands – each should be about the size of a golf ball. You'll make roughly 14–16 balls.

2 Make the tomato sauce. Heat the oil in a large casserole and fry the garlic for 1–2 minutes until just turning golden. Pour in the tomatoes and stock and season well. Simmer for about 5–8 minutes until the sauce has thickened.

3 Meanwhile, fry the meatballs. Heat the oil in a large frying pan over a low heat. Add half the meatballs and cook, turning every now and then, until golden almost all over. Transfer to a plate and then cook the other half in the same way.

4 Stir the pasta into the tomato sauce, then dot the meatballs over the top. Cover and simmer for 11 minutes over a low heat, adding the peas about 3 minutes from the end. Scatter over the lemon zest and chopped parsley to serve.

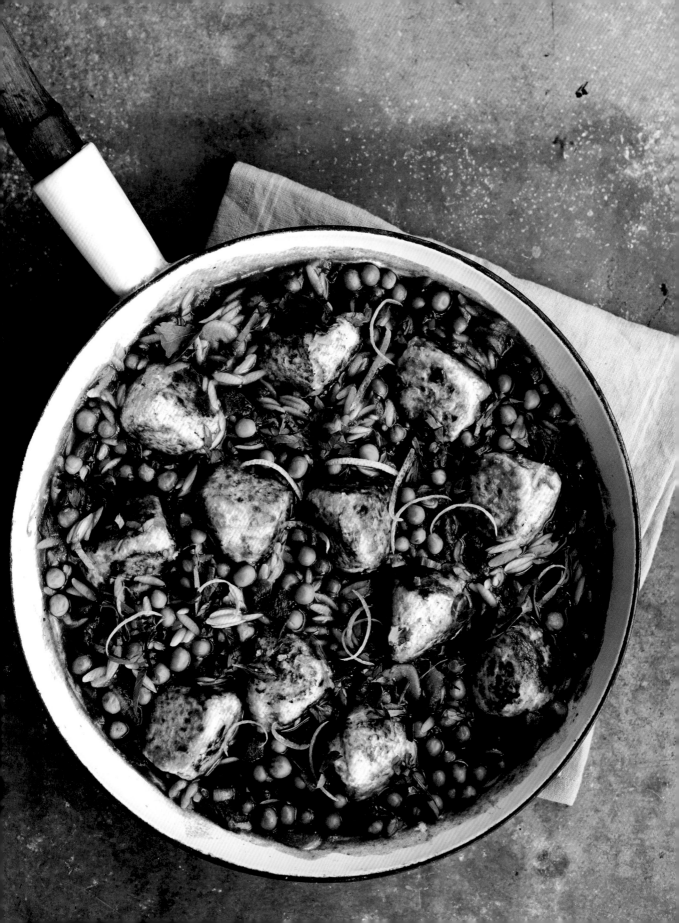

Lean lamb cutlets with beans

Lamb cutlets, trimmed of any fat, cook really quickly and are a good protein source. Serve with steamed green beans and borlotti beans, tossed with basil and a simple dressing.

SERVES 2
350 calories per serving

4 lamb cutlets, well trimmed

pinch of chilli flakes

1 tbsp olive oil

150g green beans, cut into short lengths

1 fat garlic clove, sliced

80g bag of watercress

400g can borlotti beans, drained

1 tbsp white wine vinegar

1/2 lemon, cut into wedges

sea salt and freshly ground black pepper

1 Put the lamb cutlets on a board, rub the chilli flakes over them, season with salt and pepper, then rub 1 teaspoon of the oil into them. Set aside.

2 Put the green beans into a saucepan and pour in enough water to just cover. Put a lid on the pan and bring to the boil. Cook for 3–4 minutes, or until just tender.

3 Heat a large frying pan until hot and fry the lamb over a medium-high heat for 2–3 minutes on each side. Turn off the heat and leave to rest in the pan.

4 Drain the green beans. Add the remaining oil to the saucepan and fry the sliced garlic for 1–2 minutes. Roughly chop most of the watercress. Return the green beans to the pan, add the drained borlotti beans, chopped watercress and white wine vinegar and place over a low heat. Stir well to wilt the watercress.

5 Divide the vegetables between two warm plates, top with the lamb and garnish with the remaining watercress and lemon wedges.

Teriyaki noodles with marinated tofu

Here's a simple noodle one-pot that's so tasty no one will miss the meat. You can marinate the tofu up to a day ahead, too, if you have time. Tofu is a fantastic meat alternative and is packed with protein, calcium and iron.

SERVES 2
626 calories per serving

100g soba or rice noodles

1 tbsp coconut oil, plus a little extra

1 red onion, thinly sliced

¼ savoy cabbage or 150g cavolo nero, thinly sliced

150g frozen edamame beans (soya beans)

150g chestnut mushrooms, sliced

lime wedges, to serve

For the tofu

1 tsp maple syrup

25g cashew nuts

2 tbsp teriyaki marinade

1 tbsp white wine vinegar

1cm piece of fresh root ginger, peeled and finely grated

150g firm tofu, cut into cubes

1 First marinate the tofu. Whizz the maple syrup and cashew nuts together in a small blender until the nuts are finely chopped. Stir in 1 tablespoon of the teriyaki marinade, the vinegar and ginger. Spoon into a bowl and add the tofu cubes. Toss to coat in the mixture. You can do this up to a day before if you want to get ahead – just put it into a sealable container, cover and keep in the fridge.

2 Boil the kettle and put the noodles in a large wok. Pour the boiling water over the top, to just cover, then cook according to the timings on the packet. Drain, toss with a little coconut oil to stop them from sticking and set aside.

3 Heat the tablespoon of coconut oil in the same wok, add the red onion and cook over a medium heat for 5 minutes. Add the cabbage, edamame beans (no need to defrost) and mushrooms and continue to stir-fry for 4–5 minutes until the vegetables are just tender.

4 Stir in the tofu and noodles and cook for a further 1–2 minutes until all the ingredients are hot. Divide between two bowls and serve with the lime wedges.

Spicy vegetable bean stew with giant croutons

It's very important to cook the vegetables slowly at the beginning of this recipe as this brings out the sweetness in them and gives the finished dish a really awesome flavour. The stew contains protein- and fibre-packed kidney beans, while the croutons are made by halving a bread roll and toasting until crisp, then topping with mashed avocado and feta.

SERVES 2 | plus 2 portions to freeze
373 calories per serving

2 tbsp olive oil

1 onion, finely chopped

1 red pepper, deseeded and diced

1 green pepper, deseeded and diced

½ butternut squash (about 275g), diced

1 garlic clove, sliced

½ mild red chilli, chopped

1 tsp cayenne pepper

400g can kidney beans, drained

1 tsp tomato purée

sea salt and freshly ground black pepper

To serve

1 round wholemeal roll, halved

¼ avocado

50g feta cheese, crumbled

1 Heat the oil in a large saucepan and add the onion, peppers and squash. Add a tablespoon of water and season well with salt and pepper. Stir everything together, cover with a lid and cook over a low–medium heat for 8–10 minutes, stirring every now and then, until the vegetables are softened and golden.

2 Stir in the garlic, chilli and cayenne pepper and cook for 2 minutes. Add the kidney beans, tomato purée and 250ml boiling water and bring to a simmer. Cook, uncovered, for about 10 minutes until the mixture looks like a stew. Spoon roughly half the stew into a sealable container (see Tom's Tip).

3 Preheat the grill. Toast both halves of the roll (cut sides only), under the grill until golden then mash half the avocado over each and top with the feta.

4 Divide the remaining stew between two bowls, top with the 'croutons' and serve.

TOM'S TIP

This will keep in the fridge for up to 5 days. Alternatively, freeze for up to a month. To enjoy, take out the freezer to defrost and reheat in a pan for a few minutes until hot. Add a splash of water if the stew is looking very thick.

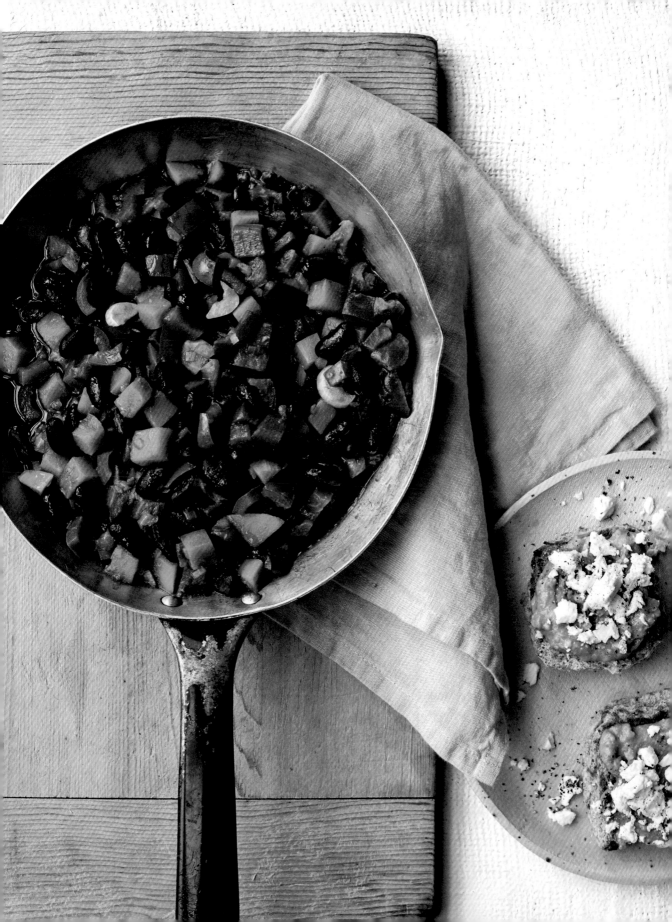

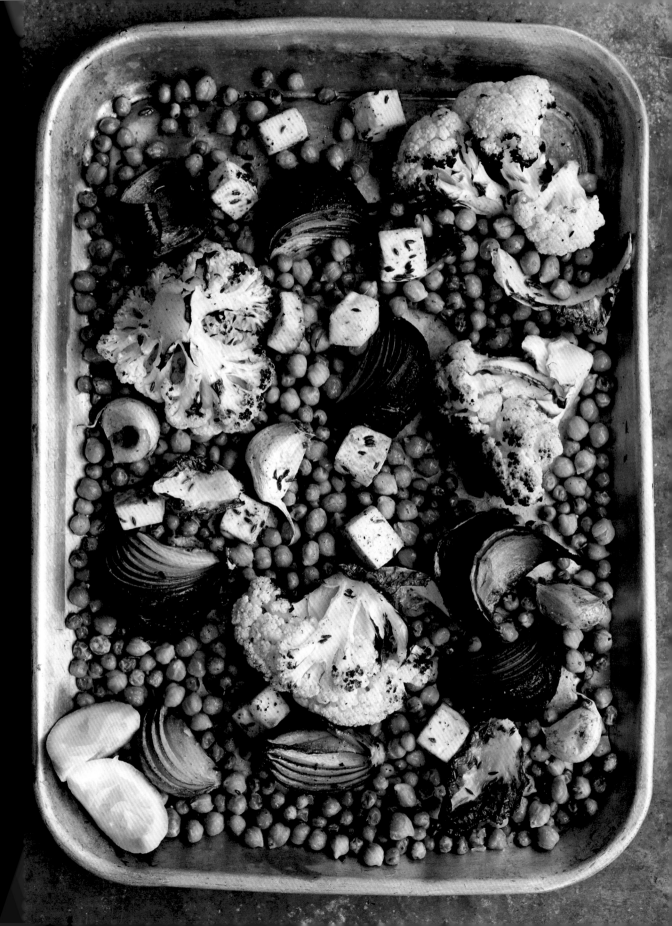

Quick-roast cauli with chickpeas & Indian spices

Tofu is delicious roasted; here it's combined with chickpeas for extra protein. The dish is enough on its own but you can also serve it with half a small naan bread per person or a small serving of brown rice if you've done a good workout.

SERVES 2
500 calories per serving

1/2 medium cauliflower, cut into 4 wedges

1 large red onion, cut into 6 wedges

100g tofu, cubed

4 garlic cloves, unpeeled

1 1/2 tbsp olive oil

1 tsp cumin seeds

1/2 tsp medium curry powder

400g can chickpeas, drained

150g frozen peas, defrosted (see Tom's Tip, page 115)

sea salt and freshly ground black pepper

To serve

1/2 lemon, cut into wedges

2 tbsp mango chutney

1 Preheat the oven to 230°C/210°C Fan/Gas 8.

2 Put the cauliflower, onion, tofu and garlic into a bowl and add 1 tablespoon of the oil, 1 tablespoon of water, the cumin seeds and curry powder. Mix well then tip into a roasting tin. Spread out in an even layer, season with salt and pepper and roast for 15–20 minutes until golden.

3 Tip the chickpeas and peas into the tin, drizzle with the remaining oil and return to the oven for 5–6 minutes, or until heated through.

4 Serve with the lemon wedges and mango chutney.

FOR A SPICY KICK I ADD HALF A CHOPPED RED CHILLI AT THE SAME TIME AS THE CHICKPEAS

weekend feasts

Whether you are catering for a crowd, or fancy making something more indulgent, my easy, creative and comforting weekend feasts will fit the bill – I've even included my one-pot roast dinner!

Chickpea korma

This homemade takeaway treat uses a ready-made korma spice paste, enriched with garlic. Serve with cucumber raita (heavy on the cucumber and light on yoghurt), some quick-to-make microwave poppadoms and a vegetable pilau. Friday night supper, done!

SERVES 2
736 calories per portion

1 tbsp coconut oil

1 tsp cumin seeds

½ cauliflower, chopped

75g peas (fresh or frozen)

100g brown basmati rice

2–3 tbsp ready-made korma paste, depending on how spicy you like it

2 garlic cloves, crushed

1 tbsp tomato purée

2 tbsp ground almonds

400g can chickpeas, drained

3 tbsp Greek yoghurt

15g coriander leaves

15g flaked almonds, toasted (optional)

sea salt and freshly ground black pepper

To serve

10cm piece of cucumber, grated

2 uncooked poppadoms

1 Heat half the coconut oil in a saucepan over a medium heat and add the cumin seeds. When they start to sizzle, add the cauliflower and peas and stir-fry for 2–3 minutes. Add the rice to the pan and pour in 350ml boiling water. Cover with a lid, turn the heat down to low, and cook for 25 minutes until the rice is tender.

2 Heat the remaining oil in a separate saucepan and add the korma paste and garlic. Add 2 tablespoons of water and the tomato purée and stir over a medium heat until the mixture looks like a paste. Stir in another 2 tablespoons of water, two more times, until the mixture has thickened and looks slightly less oily. Stir in the ground almonds and chickpeas and cook for 1 minute.

3 Pour 250–300ml boiling water into the pan, season well and cover the pan with a lid. Simmer for about 15 minutes, then turn off the heat and stir in half the yoghurt.

4 Stir the cucumber and remaining yoghurt together in a small bowl. Microwave the poppadoms following the instructions on the packet.

5 When the rice is ready, fluff up with a fork. Divide between two bowls and top with the chickpea curry. Scatter over the coriander and flaked almonds, if using. Serve with the cucumber raita and poppadoms.

TOM'S TIP

For a vegan version of this, use a non-dairy yoghurt in the korma and raita.

One-pot gammon with roots

This everything-in-the-pot recipe provides enough food for not just one meal but three! Serve the gammon sliced and hot with the vegetables, and then use the leftovers in the Pea & Ham Soup (see page 95), sliced in a sandwich or shredded on top of a Tartine (see page 99). You can also use the reserved cooked leek and potato and the stock in the Pea & Ham Soup recipe.

SERVES 4, WITH LEFTOVERS
382 calories per portion

1.4kg unsmoked gammon joint

300ml cider

1 litre hot vegetable stock

few sprigs of thyme (optional)

2 fat garlic cloves, unpeeled

1 large leek (about 280g), chopped into 6 chunks

6 Chantenay carrots, halved

225g swede, peeled and cut into large chunks

8 new potatoes (225g), halved

8 stems of tenderstem or purple sprouting broccoli

15g butter, softened

15g plain flour

15g parsley, finely chopped

sea salt and freshly ground black pepper

1 Put the gammon into a large casserole with the cider, hot stock, thyme, if using, and garlic. Cover the pan with a lid and bring to a simmer. Turn the heat down low, so the liquid is gently simmering and cook for 1 hour.

2 Add the leek, carrots, swede and new potatoes and continue to simmer for 25 minutes. Add the broccoli and cook for a further 4–5 minutes until the broccoli is cooked but still tender.

3 Lift the gammon and vegetables on to a warm platter, cover with foil to keep warm and set aside. Whip out and discard the thyme and reserve the garlic. Strain 300ml of the stock into a jug and the remainder into a container and set aside.

4 Mash the butter and flour together in a small bowl and season well. Squeeze the cooked garlic out of its skin and mash briefly on a board, then put into the casserole with the 300ml reserved stock. Bring the stock to a simmer and whisk in the butter and flour mixture. Simmer for 3–5 minutes, whisking all the time, until the stock thickens slightly. Stir in the chopped parsley.

5 Slice the cooked gammon joint, giving each person 2–3 slices (125–150g) with a piece of leek and three potato halves. Divvy up the carrots, swede and broccoli. Spoon over the parsley sauce and serve.

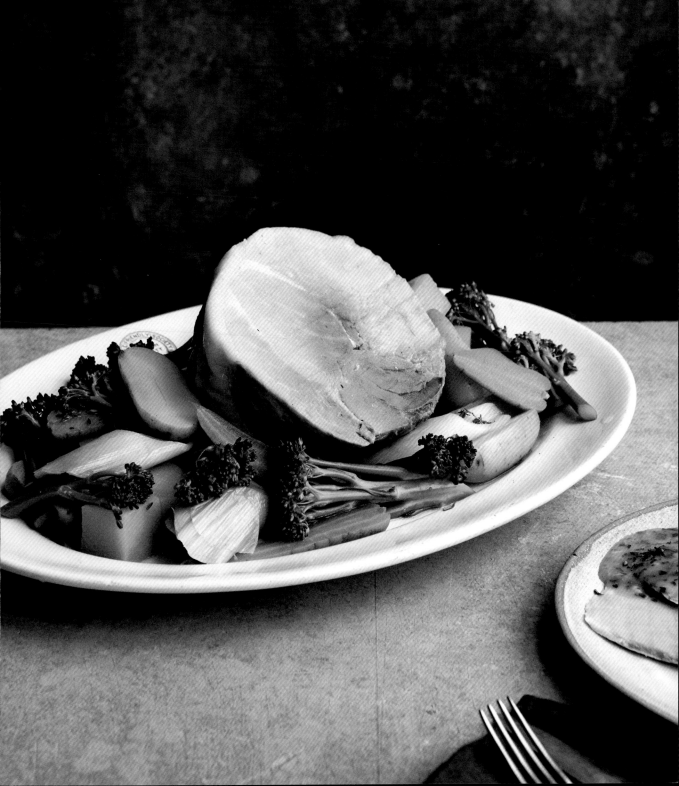

One-pot sort of Sunday roast for two

Here's a great way to do a healthy Sunday 'roast' with all the flavour and goodness but fewer calories. Layer everything up in one big pan, pour in stock and let the oven do all the work.

SERVES 2
511 calories per portion

2 chicken leg quarters (thigh and drumstick)

1 tsp olive oil

1 sausage, twisted and cut in half

1/2 medium onion, cut into 4 wedges

1 large carrot, cut into 4 chunks

4 small parsnips, halved or cut into chunks

175g turnip, cut into chunks

2–3 sprigs of thyme, plus extra leaves to garnish

450ml light chicken stock

150g frozen peas, defrosted (see Tom's Tip, page 115)

1 Preheat the oven to 180°C/160°C Fan/Gas 4.

2 Heat a large casserole until hot and add the chicken pieces skin side down. Cook for 1–2 minutes, then drizzle in the oil. Continue to cook over a low-medium heat until the skin is browned on one side. Flip over and cook the other side until seared. At the same time, brown the halved sausage. Lift them out on to a plate and set aside.

3 Add the onion and chunks of carrot, parsnip and turnip and spread out over the base of the casserole. Continue to cook over a low heat for 8–10 minutes until golden.

4 Tuck the thyme around the vegetables then pour in the stock. Return the chicken and sausages to the casserole, cover with a lid and place in the oven for 1 hour.

5 When the hour is up, add the peas and return to the oven for 10 minutes to heat through. Serve with a few fresh thyme leaves over the top.

Veggie Bolognese

Batch cooking at the weekend is an easy way to make a feast for a weekday supper – this recipe makes 6 portions. Vegetarian mince and lentils provide extra protein and fibre.

SERVES 2 | PLUS 4 PORTIONS TO FREEZE
447 calories per portion

1 tbsp olive oil

1 onion, chopped

2 garlic cloves, sliced

150g chestnut mushrooms, finely chopped

350g vegetarian mince

100g red lentils

pinch of chilli flakes

sprig of thyme

400g can chopped tomatoes

600ml hot vegetable stock

sea salt and freshly ground black pepper

To serve

150g tagliatelle or fettuccine pasta

10g Parmesan cheese

1 Heat the oil in a large saucepan and stir in the chopped onion, along with 2 tablespoons of boiling water. Season well and cook, stirring occasionally, over a low–medium heat for about 8 minutes, or until the onion has turned golden and started to soften.

2 Stir in the garlic and mushrooms and continue to cook, stirring regularly, for about 5 minutes until the mushrooms have cooked through.

3 Stir in the mince and lentils and add a good shake of chilli flakes, depending on how spicy you like it. Add the thyme sprig to the pan with the tomatoes and stock. Stir everything again then cover the pan with a lid and bring to a simmer. Cook over a low heat for 30 minutes, stirring every now and then.

4 About 10 minutes before the sauce is ready, bring a large saucepan of salted water to the boil. Add the pasta and cook according to the timings on the packet. Drain, leaving about 2 tablespoons of water in the pan, then return the pasta to the pan.

5 When the sauce is ready, scoop two-thirds of it into a sealable container for another day (see Tom's Tip). Stir the remaining sauce into the pasta pan until it is all coated and divide between two bowls. Grate the Parmesan and serve.

TOM'S TIP

Divide the remaining sauce in half and freeze in two separate containers. Cover, label and freeze. To enjoy next time round, defrost overnight and reheat in a pan until hot all the way through.

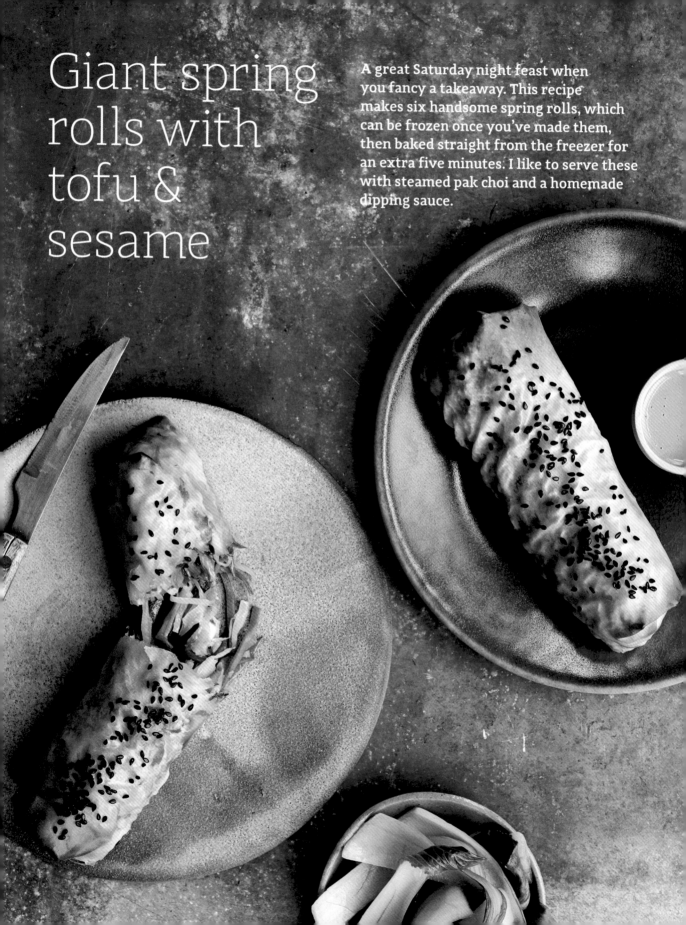

Giant spring rolls with tofu & sesame

A great Saturday night feast when you fancy a takeaway. This recipe makes six handsome spring rolls, which can be frozen once you've made them, then baked straight from the freezer for an extra five minutes. I like to serve these with steamed pak choi and a homemade dipping sauce.

2 tsp coconut oil

6 spring onions, thinly sliced

2 garlic cloves, sliced

2cm piece of fresh root ginger, peeled and sliced into matchsticks

2 carrots (about 350g), shredded

100g mangetout or sugar snap peas, chopped lengthways into 3 or 4 slices

100g baby corn, sliced

1/2 medium white cabbage, shredded

about 125g firm tofu, diced

1 tbsp soy sauce

1 tbsp olive oil

270g packet (7 sheets) of filo pastry (see tip below)

2 tsp black sesame seeds

2 large pak choi, leaves separated

For the dipping sauce

1 tsp maple syrup

2 tsp peanut butter

1 tbsp soy sauce

1/2 tsp tomato purée

1 Melt the coconut oil in a large wok or saucepan over a medium heat and add the spring onions, garlic, ginger, carrots, mangetout (or sugar snaps), corn and cabbage, along with a tablespoon of water. Stir-fry for 12–15 minutes until the vegetables have cooked down and softened – they'll have wilted to about half their volume and be turning a bit golden. Stir in the tofu and soy sauce, then spoon into a bowl and set aside to cool.

2 Pour the olive oil into a small glass, add 2 tablespoons of water and whisk together. Preheat the oven to 200°C/180°C Fan/Gas 6.

3 Lay a sheet of pastry on a board then double it over to make into a square. Spoon about a sixth of the mixture on to the pastry in a horizontal line in the middle, leaving a 2cm border along the edges.

4 Fold the top over so it half covers the cooked vegetables, then tuck the sides in too and roll the pastry bundle down to wrap up the filling. When you almost reach the bottom, tuck the lower edge under to neaten, brush with the oil and water mixture and fold in to

complete the parcel. Turn over so the seam is on the other side.

5 Brush the top with the oil mixture, sprinkle with a few sesame seeds and put on a baking sheet. Repeat with the remaining filo sheets and filling to make six spring rolls.

6 Bake for 20 minutes until crisp and golden. Meanwhile, make the sauce by stirring together the maple syrup, peanut butter, soy sauce, tomato purée and 1/2 tablespoon of boiling water in a small bowl – add 1–2 teaspoons more water if it's very thick.

7 Steam the pak choi in a saucepan with a couple of tablespoons of water for a few minutes, or until tender.

8 Serve each spring roll with the pak choi and some dipping sauce drizzled over the top.

TOM'S TIP

A packet of 7 sheets of pastry will leave one sheet for Berry Parcels (see page 174). Wrap it in cling film, label and freeze for up to a month. Remove from the freezer an hour before using.

Roast chicken with vegetable bake

This is a great crowd-pleasing roast chicken recipe, which is served on top of an easy vegetable bake. Serve with steamed greens or salad and, if you have some very hungry mouths to feed, a bowl of lightly buttered new potatoes (see Tom's Tip).

SERVES 6
470 calories per portion

1 whole chicken, about 1.5–1.8kg

1¹/₂ tbsp olive oil

sea salt and freshly ground black pepper

For the bake

1 large aubergine, cut into 5mm slices

250g butternut squash, peeled or unpeeled and sliced

2 peppers, deseeded and halved

2 tbsp olive oil

2 garlic cloves, crushed

400g can chopped tomatoes

175g ricotta cheese

1 medium egg

10g Parmesan cheese, grated

1 Preheat the oven to 220°C/200°C Fan/Gas 7.

2 Put the chicken into a roasting tin, drizzle with the oil and season well. Pour 300ml cold water into the tin.

3 Line a separate roasting tin with baking parchment and add the sliced aubergine, squash and peppers in a single layer. Mix 1 tablespoon of the oil with 2 tablespoons of water, season well and pour over the veg.

4 Transfer both the chicken and the vegetables to the oven, with the chicken sitting on the upper shelf, and roast for 20 minutes. Reduce the oven temperature to 190°C/170°C Fan/Gas 5 and continue to roast for 1 hour.

5 About 20 minutes before the end of the cooking time, heat the remaining olive oil in a saucepan and stir in the garlic. Cook for 1–2 minutes then add the chopped tomatoes and 100ml water. Season well, bring to a simmer and bubble for 10 minutes.

A BIG BOWL OF GREENS ON THE SIDE IS A MUST WITH THIS RECIPE! I LIKE TO STEAM KALE – IT'S PACKED WITH VITAMINS A, C AND K

6 Remove the roasted vegetables from the oven and transfer to an ovenproof dish. Spoon the tomato sauce over the top. Beat the ricotta and egg together in a bowl and season well. Dollop spoonfuls of this mixture over the tomato sauce, then scatter the grated Parmesan over the top.

7 Take the chicken out of the oven, then put the vegetable bake into the oven for 15 minutes to heat through and cook the ricotta mixture.

8 Pour the juices from the chicken into a bowl. Cover the chicken in foil and set aside to rest. Skim off the fat from the juices with a spoon, then pour the remaining juices into a pan and simmer for 10 minutes until reduced by about two-thirds. Pour into a jug.

9 Carve the chicken into slices and serve with the vegetable bake and the juices poured over.

TOM'S TIP
To serve this with new potatoes, allow 150g per person, halved or quartered. Add to a pan of boiling water and simmer for 15 minutes until very tender. Drain, return to the pan with 10g butter and seasoning, then shake to coat the potatoes.

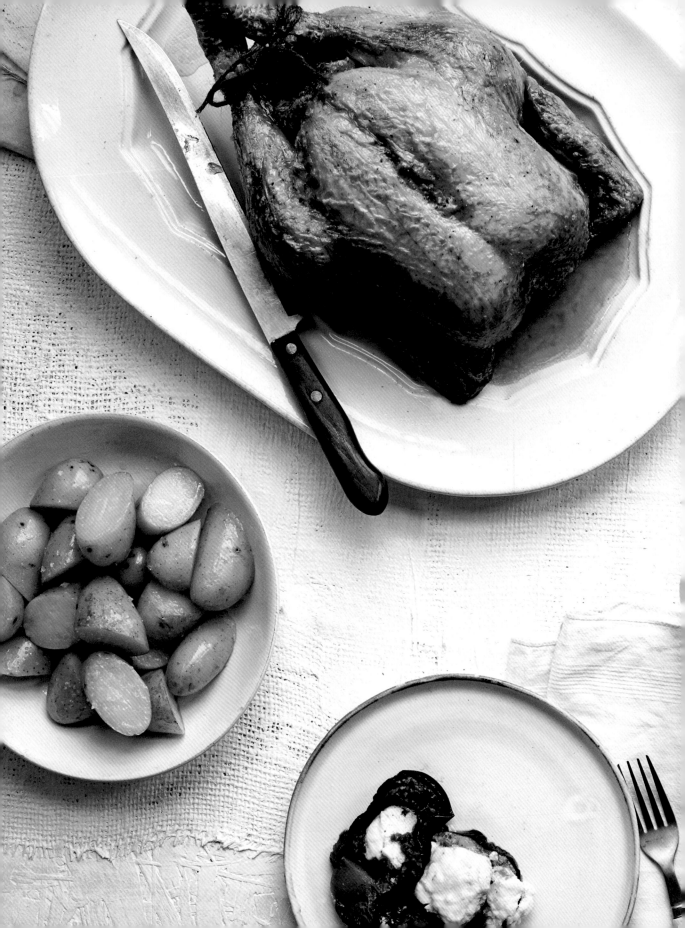

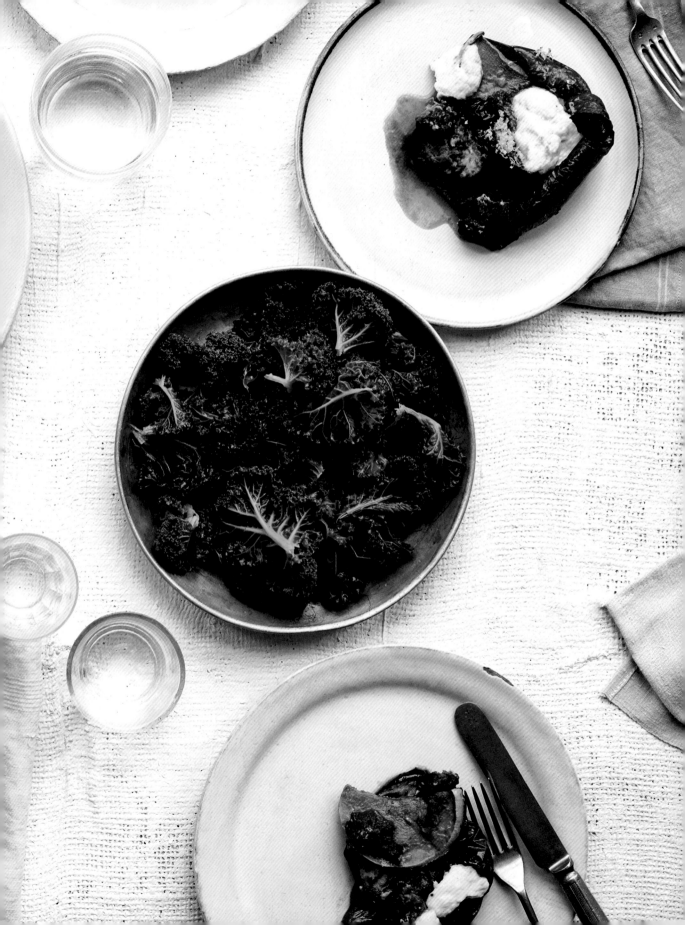

Tom's Olympic burger

Yes, burgers can be healthy – if you cut the chips and serve with a crisp salad on the side. This one is packed with an extra portion of protein in the form of an egg and I've swapped the mayo for a cheesy spring onion dip to serve alongside or dollop on the wholemeal bun.

SERVES 2
792 calories per serving

250g minced beef

3 sprigs of thyme

1 tsp smoked paprika

1 tsp olive oil, plus extra for drizzling

2 medium eggs

2 wholemeal burger buns, split

2 baby gem lettuces, halved

2 tomatoes on the vine, quartered

sea salt and freshly ground black pepper

For the dip

2 spring onions, chopped

2 tbsp Greek yoghurt

50g Cheddar cheese or blue cheese

1 First make the dip: put the spring onions, yoghurt and cheese into a mini blender with 2 tablespoons of cold water and season well. Blitz to make a smooth dip and spoon into a bowl.

2 Put the mince into a bowl and add the thyme and paprika. Season well and mix everything together then divide the mixture roughly in half.

3 Take one portion and shape on a board into a large round, flat patty, around 1cm thick. Carefully push your finger through the middle to make a hole. Keep pushing the mince out until you've made a hole in the middle about 6cm in diameter. Flatten the patty again slightly. Do the same with the rest of the mixture so you've made two burgers.

4 Heat the oil in a large frying pan and slide the burgers into it. Cook for 2–3 minutes on one side, until golden, then flip each one over. Crack an egg into each hole and continue to cook for 4–5 minutes, covered, until the egg is set.

5 Put a burger bun base on to each plate and drizzle with about 1/2 teaspoon of oil (toast them first if you want to). Divide the lettuce and tomatoes between the plates too.

6 Carefully lift the burgers on to each bun and top with the other bun half. Serve with the cheese and onion dip.

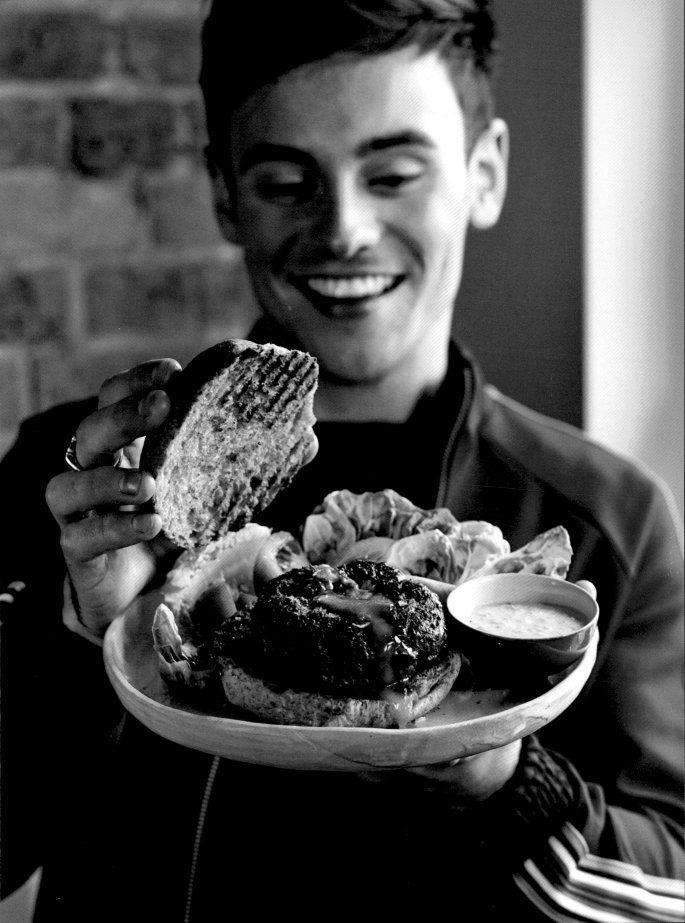

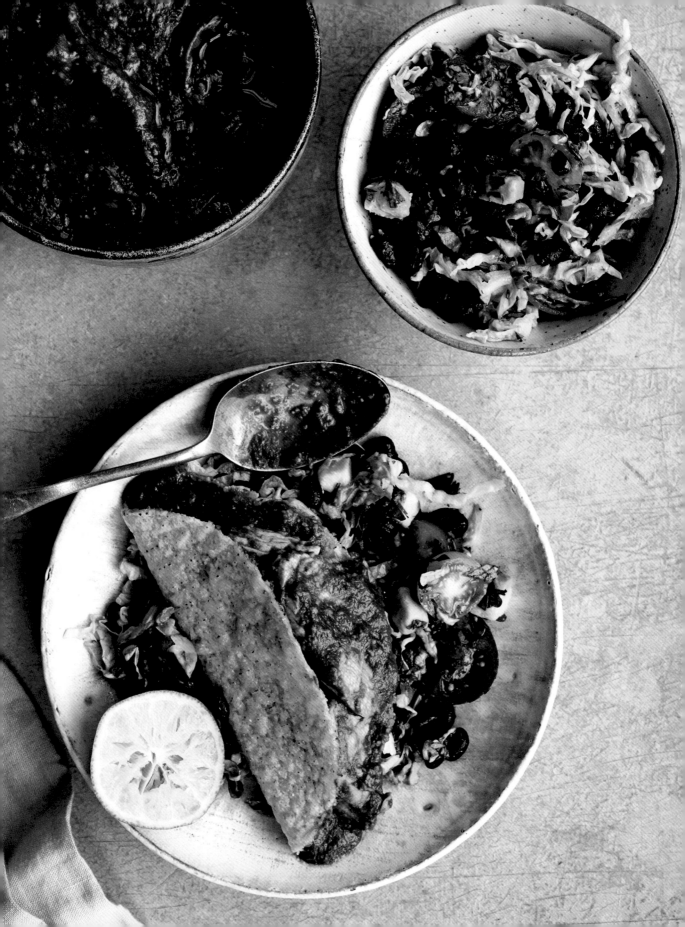

Cheat's turkey mole

This recipe makes a base sauce – the mole – that is enough for 6 portions. I've given instructions to use some of the sauce to make a delicious and healthy meal for two. Pack the remaining sauce into freezerproof containers or bags and freeze to use another time.

SERVES 2 |
PLUS 4 PORTIONS TO FREEZE
554 calories per portion

For the base

1 onion, chopped

1 garlic clove, chopped

1/2 tsp chilli flakes

1/2 tsp ground cinnamon

1 tsp cayenne pepper

25g unsalted peanuts

1 tbsp olive oil

25g raisins

400g can chopped tomatoes

400ml hot chicken stock

15g dark chocolate (at least 85% cocoa solids)

sea salt and freshly ground black pepper

To serve

300g turkey breast steaks, cut into strips

400g can black beans, drained

200g yellow and red cherry tomatoes, halved

2 tbsp chopped coriander

1/2 avocado, chopped

1/2 small iceberg lettuce or 2 little gems, shredded

2 taco shells

1 lime, cut into wedges

1 Put a frying pan over a medium heat and add the onion, garlic, chilli flakes, cinnamon, cayenne and peanuts. Cook for 1–2 minutes to slightly brown the onion and toast the spices in the heat of the pan.

2 Drizzle in the olive oil and 2 tablespoons of water and continue to cook the onion, spices and nuts for 10 minutes until starting to soften. Stir in the raisins and chopped tomatoes and pour in the stock. Bring to a simmer then cook for 15 minutes over a low-medium heat. Stir in the chocolate and let it melt. Allow to cool a little, then purée with a stick blender. Spoon two-thirds of the sauce into two separate containers to freeze for another day.

3 Season the sauce, then add the turkey strips to the pan and bring to a simmer. Cover with a lid and cook for 10–15 minutes, or until the turkey is tender.

4 While the turkey is cooking, put the beans into a bowl, add the tomatoes, coriander, avocado and lettuce and mix together. Season well.

5 Spoon the turkey mole between the taco shells and serve with the bean salsa and lime wedges.

Crunchy chicken & sweet potato chips

Here's my version of chicken and chips. Both are cooked in the oven for a slightly healthier take on the classic. Serve with a wholesome portion of peas.

SERVES 2
644 calories per portion

2 x 150g skinless chicken breasts

75ml milk

2 tbsp plain flour or cornflour

1 medium egg

40g lightly salted tortilla chips (see page 170 for a tip to use up leftover tortilla chips)

1/2–1 tsp fajita spice mix, depending on how hot you like it

150g frozen peas

sea salt and freshly ground black pepper

For the sweet potato chips

2 sprigs of thyme

2 sweet potatoes (about 350g), unpeeled, cut into chips

1¹/2 tsp olive oil

1 Preheat the oven to 200°C/180°C Fan/Gas 6.

2 Put the chicken into a small container and pour over the milk. Set aside for at least 30 minutes to tenderise the chicken. If you have time, you can chill this in the fridge up to a day ahead.

3 Meanwhile, strip the leaves off the thyme sprigs and put in a bowl with the sweet potatoes and olive oil. Season well and toss together, then spread out on a baking sheet.

4 Put the flour or cornflour into a bowl and beat the egg in another. Whizz the tortilla chips and fajita spice mix in a mini blender until the crisps look like crumbs and tip into a third bowl.

5 Lift one of the chicken breasts out of the milk and dip first into the flour mixture, then the egg and finally the tortilla crumbs, pressing gently to coat. Do the same with the other piece. Put on a non-stick baking sheet.

6 Transfer both the chicken and sweet potato chips to the oven and bake for 25–30 minutes.

7 About 5 minutes before the chicken and sweet potatoes are ready, bring a small pan of water to the boil. Add the frozen peas (no need to defrost) and cook for 2–3 minutes until tender. Drain well.

8 Divide the chicken, sweet potatoes and peas between two plates and serve.

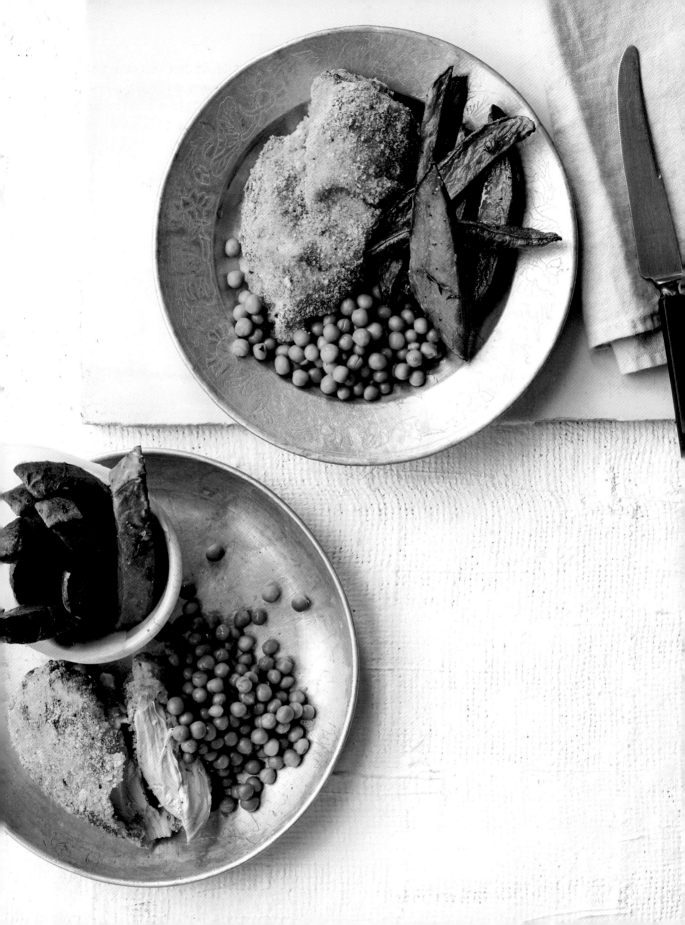

Aubergine & sweet potato cake

This savoury cake is like a frittata, the Italian vegetable bake set with eggs. Aubergine, sweet potatoes and peppers are grilled until tender then layered up in a cake tin. A mixture of beaten eggs, whizzed together with feta cheese and parsley is poured over the top, then breadcrumbs, feta and nuts are scattered on top and the whole lot is baked until golden. This is very filling and nourishing thanks to the vegetables and good proteins here – just serve with a crisp green salad or steamed greens on the side.

SERVES 6
238 calories per portion

1 tbsp olive oil, plus extra for greasing

3 peppers, halved and deseeded

2 aubergines, sliced into 1–2cm rounds

3 sweet potatoes (about 500g), sliced into 2cm rounds

3 medium eggs, beaten

100g feta cheese, crumbled

15g chopped parsley

15g white or wholemeal breadcrumbs

10g pine nuts

sea salt and freshly ground black pepper

1 Preheat the grill. Grease a 20cm deep cake tin and line with baking parchment.

2 Arrange the peppers on a baking sheet and grill until the skin has blistered and blackened slightly. Tip into a bowl and cover with a lid or a large plate to steam the skins off the peppers. Once cool, peel off and discard the skins.

3 Brush the oil all over the aubergine and sweet potato slices and grill in batches on the baking sheet until golden and tender.

4 Preheat the oven to 200°C/180°C Fan/Gas 6.

5 Put the eggs, half the feta cheese and the parsley into the bowl of a food processor and season well. Whizz until smooth.

6 Layer the grilled vegetables up in the tin, starting with the sweet potatoes and peppers and finishing with a layer of aubergines. Pour the egg mixture all over the vegetables, then scatter over the remaining feta, the breadcrumbs and pine nuts. Bake in the oven for 25–30 minutes until golden on top.

7 Leave to sit in the tin for 10 minutes, then remove from the tin and serve sliced into wedges.

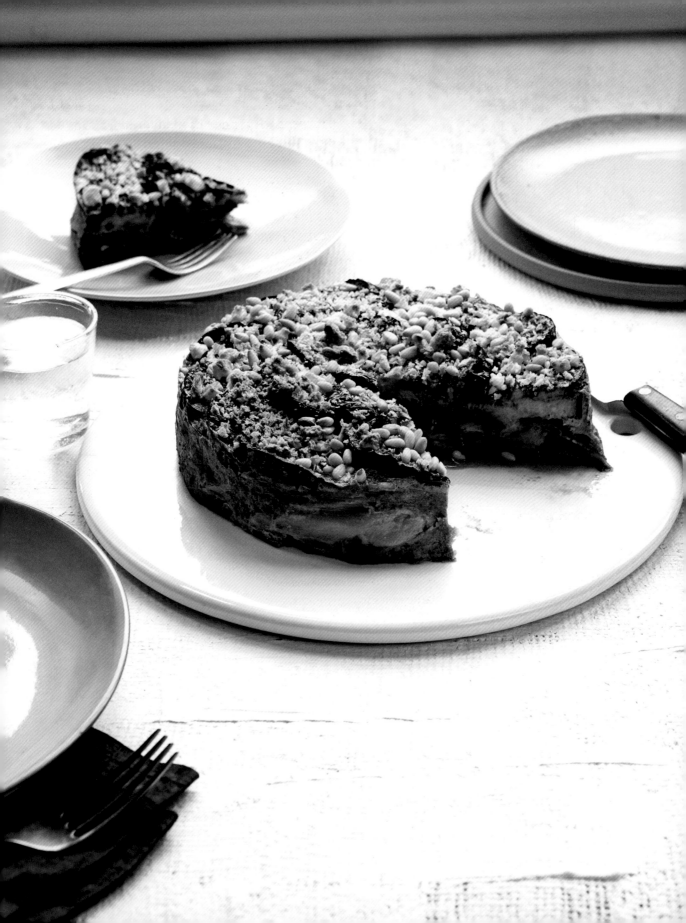

Sausage & smash

It's really quite simple to make your own healthy sausages if you roll them in something that will help to keep their barrel shape. These have a lovely coating of oats, which gives them a slight crunch.

SERVES 2
436 calories per portion

250g skinless chicken thigh fillets

zest of 1 lemon

25g sultanas

25g oats

2 tsp olive oil

sea salt and freshly ground black pepper

lemon quarters, to serve

For the 'smash'

300g new potatoes, quartered

150g frozen broad beans, peas or mixed vegetables

15g chopped parsley, plus a few leaves to garnish

5g butter

1 Preheat the oven to 220°C/200°C Fan/Gas 7.

2 Put the chicken into a food processor and add the lemon zest and plenty of salt and pepper. Whizz until the chicken is finely chopped. Add the sultanas and whizz again to briefly combine.

3 Divide into four equal portions and roll each one into a sausage, then roll in the oats. Put on a baking sheet, drizzle each with about 1/2 teaspoon of oil and bake in the oven for 20 minutes.

4 Bring a medium saucepan of water to the boil and add the potatoes. Bring to a simmer and cook for 12 minutes, then add the frozen vegetables to the pan (no need to defrost). Once the potatoes are tender, drain well and return to the pan. Add the parsley and butter to the pan and mash well.

5 Divide the smash between two plates and top with the sausages and serve with a few parsley leaves and the lemon quarters on the side.

SWEET POTATOES MAKE REALLY GOOD MASH TOO

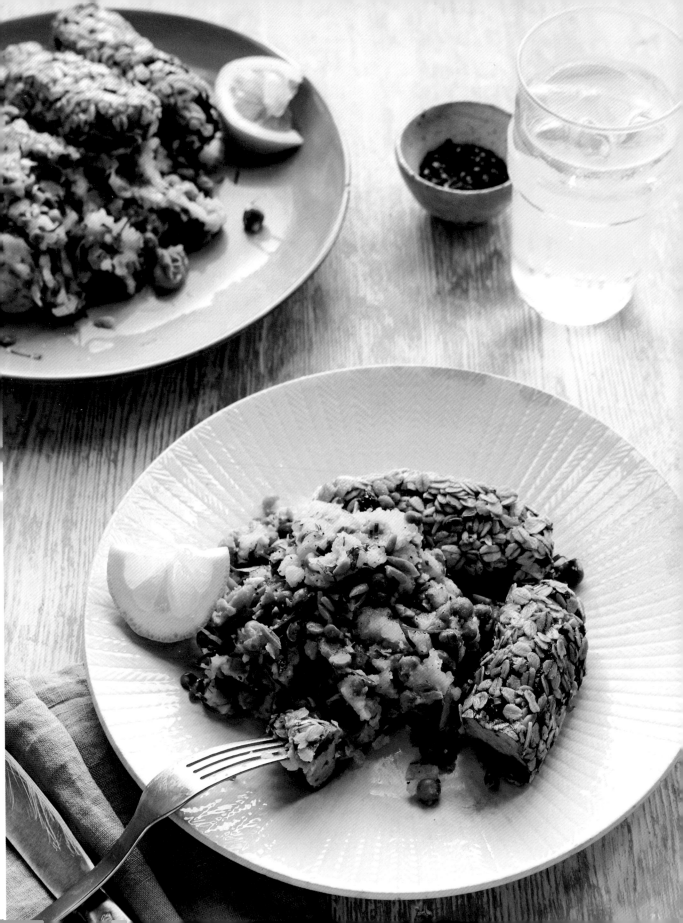

My all-the-veg pasta bake

There are all sorts of gluten-free pastas available now in supermarkets so I experimented with one of them for this recipe. Green pea pasta is made from green pea flour and is higher in fibre and protein than traditional pasta. It tastes great in this and makes a really colourful addition. Check out my tip below, too – it tastes awesome!

Serves 4–6
472 calories per portion

1 tbsp olive oil

2 garlic cloves, chopped

1 red onion, roughly chopped

1 red pepper, deseeded and chopped

1 yellow pepper, deseeded and chopped

400g butternut squash, peeled or unpeeled and chopped

400g can chopped tomatoes

600ml hot vegetable stock

250g green pea fusilli pasta

2 sprigs of basil, leaves roughly chopped

2 x 125g balls of mozzarella, roughly chopped

sea salt and freshly ground black pepper

1 Heat the oil in a large saucepan and add the garlic, onion, peppers and squash. Season well and pour in 2 tablespoons of water. Cover with a lid and cook over a low-medium heat for 10–12 minutes until the vegetables start to soften.

2 Stir in the chopped tomatoes and stock and bring to a simmer. Cover with a lid and cook over a medium heat for 15 minutes. The sauce should have reduced down and not be too liquid after this time. If there's a lot of extra liquid in the pan, take the lid off and simmer over a medium-high heat for 5 minutes to reduce it.

3 Preheat the oven to 200°C/180°C Fan/Gas 6. Meanwhile, bring a large pan of salted water to the boil and cook the pasta for 6 minutes, or according to the timings on the packet.

4 Drain the pasta and return to the pan, then spoon the vegetable sauce on top along with the basil. Season with pepper and stir everything together. Spoon into a large 1.5–2 litre ovenproof dish.

5 Scatter the mozzarella over the top and bake in the oven for 20–25 minutes until golden on top.

TOM'S TIP
One of my favourite ways to top a pasta bake is with tortilla chips – but only if I have a small packet to hand or already have one open. You'll need about 50g to top this bake – just crunch them up into bits before sprinkling over the top.

Braised beef with beans & roasted broccoli

I've used beef short rib for this recipe as cooking meat on the bone gives it lots more flavour. There's very little prep here – so it's great for a lazy Sunday – then it just needs about 3 hours in the oven for the beef to become really tender and very tasty. Serve with roasted broccoli.

Serves 4
473 calories per portion

1 tbsp olive oil

4 x beef short ribs (about 1kg)

12 shallots

4 garlic cloves, unpeeled

1 red or green mild chilli, halved lengthways

450g hot beef stock

2 x 400g cans mixed beans, drained

300g tenderstem broccoli

15g chopped parsley

sea salt and freshly ground black pepper

1 Preheat the oven to 170°C/150°C Fan/Gas 2.

2 Heat 2 teaspoons of the oil in a large casserole. Season the beef and brown each piece over a low–medium heat until each side is really dark. The darker the colour, the better the flavour will be.

3 Put on a plate while you brown the shallots. They won't need any more oil and will brown quite quickly as the casserole will already be really hot. Add the garlic cloves and chilli and return the beef to the casserole. Pour in the stock, season well and cover with a lid. Transfer to the oven to cook for 3 hours.

4 About half an hour before the beef is ready, stir in the drained mixed beans. Add a splash more hot water if you feel it needs more liquid.

5 Spread the broccoli out on a roasting tin and brush with the remaining oil. Season well. Roast on a shelf below the casserole for 20–25 minutes, or until tender.

6 When the beef is very tender, strip the meat off the bones and discard them. Lift out the garlic cloves at the same time. Squeeze them out of their papery skins, roughly mash and return to the pan. Roughly shred the beef and stir back into the stew, along with the parsley. Spoon into bowls and serve with the roasted broccoli.

TOM'S TIP

I've served this with roasted broccoli but if you like an extra side, bake some small sweet potatoes on a baking sheet for 1 hour on a shelf below the casserole.

desserts & drinks

From millionaire shortbread puds, through to my dead easy ice cream, these dessert and drink options will ensure you finish off your meal in style!

The anytime smoothie

The addition of protein powder here makes this a perfect post-workout smoothie. It's also great for breakfast, topped with a spoonful of yoghurt and chopped fruit.

SERVES 2
249 calories per serving

75g spinach

1 tbsp cacao powder

1/2 banana, chopped

2 soft ready-to-eat dates

25g almond butter

10g unsweetened plain protein powder

10g oats

1 tsp honey (optional)

1 Put the spinach into the bowl of a food processor or high-speed blender. Add the cacao powder, banana, dates, almond butter, protein powder, oats and honey, if using.

2 Whizz everything together until combined, then pour in 125ml water and whizz again until smooth.

3 Pour into a glass and serve.

Virgin orange mojito

This is a refreshing iced drink, laced with orange and mint. Oranges are packed with vitamin C and potassium to boost immunity and heart health. The antioxidants in cinnamon also have an anti-inflammatory effect.

SERVES 2
50 calories per serving

1 tsp honey

1/2 tsp ground cinnamon

juice of 3 large oranges

2 tbsp finely chopped mint, plus 2 sprigs to decorate

ice

1 Put the honey and cinnamon into a small jug. Add 1–2 tablespoons of boiling water and mix together, then set aside to cool.

2 Stir in the orange juice and chopped mint.

3 Fill two glasses with ice, pour the mojito over the top and decorate each with a sprig of mint.

Piña colada smoothie

If you're having a party but don't want to drink alcohol, this lower-calorie take on the summer classic, made with pineapple, coconut, yoghurt and lime is one to beat. Even without the rum, you will feel like you are sitting on a warm beach somewhere tropical!

SERVES 2
160 calories per serving

250g chopped fresh pineapple

100g natural yoghurt or coconut yoghurt

zest and juice of 1 small ripe lime

20g unsweetened desiccated coconut

6 ice cubes

1 Put the pineapple into the bowl of a food processor. Add the yoghurt, lime zest and juice, desiccated coconut and 4 of the ice cubes.

2 Whizz until the pineapple is blended and the ice is roughly crushed to make a smoothie.

3 Divide between two glasses, top each with one more ice cube and serve.

Berry parcels with a chocolate sauce

These parcels are a little fiddly to make as there isn't a lot of pastry to play with, but once you've tried them you'll love them. The thin layer of crisp pastry means they're lighter than a traditional pudding so I've served these with a rich chocolate sauce to drizzle over. And the recipe is easy to multiply if you're serving more people. Serve this straight away, as the pastry is quite delicate.

SERVES 2

167 calories per serving

2 tsp sunflower or olive oil

1 sheet of filo pastry

80g frozen summer fruits

good pinch of unrefined caster sugar

15g dark chocolate (at least 70% cocoa solids)

1 tbsp maple syrup

TOM'S TIP
Use the remaining filo sheets to make my Giant Spring Rolls (see page 154).

1 Preheat the oven to 200°C/180°C Fan/Gas 6. Mix the sunflower oil and 2 teaspoons of cold water in a glass.

2 Cut the sheet of filo in half to make two squares. Take one square and put it on a board. Spoon half the fruits into the bottom left-hand corner of the pastry, leaving a 5cm border at each edge. Fold the pastry up at the bottom then in from the left to partly cover the fruit. Keeping the fruit in the corner of the pastry, fold the filled corner over so that the fruit is wrapped in the pastry and shaped like a triangle.

3 Fold the top piece of unfilled pastry over the top to cover the fruit with another layer of pastry. Then fold the other piece of pastry on top to cover, folding it round and underneath the parcel. You'll have made a triangular parcel at this stage.

4 Brush the oil mixture all over to secure all the ends and stick the pastry down. Transfer to a baking sheet. Do the same with the other piece of pastry and place on the baking sheet, too. Sprinkle each parcel with a pinch of sugar

5 Bake in the oven for 8–10 minutes until golden. About 5 minutes before the parcels have finished baking, put the dark chocolate and maple syrup into a small bowl with 1 tablespoon of water. Melt in a microwave at the lowest power setting for about 3 minutes, stirring occasionally. Whisk together to make a smooth sauce.

6 Put each of the parcels on a plate and serve while still hot with the sauce.

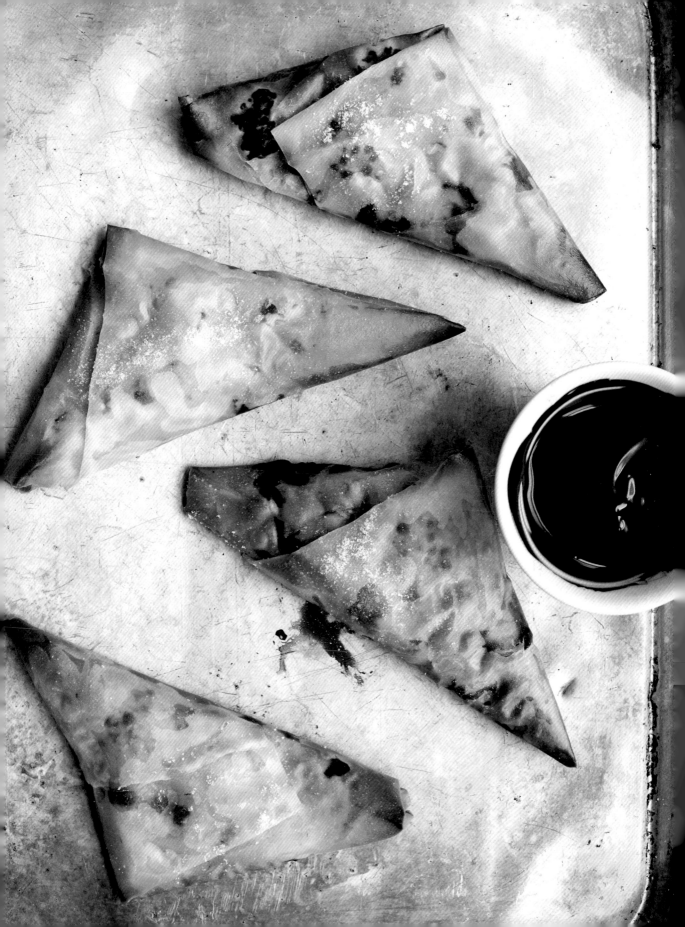

Tom's dead easy banana ice cream trio

Keep chopped banana in the freezer and then whizz to make a soft-scoop ice cream whenever you fancy a treat, adding other ingredients according to whichever flavours you like. Once the banana has been blended, it softens and starts to melt so if you want to firm it up, just pop it in the freezer for half an hour. All serve 2.

Cinnamon

86 calories per serving

1 tsp ground coffee

1 tsp vanilla extract

1/2 tsp ground cinnamon

2 bananas, chopped and frozen until firm

1 Put the coffee, vanilla extract and cinnamon into a small glass and pour over a tablespoon of boiling water. Stir to dissolve then let it cool.
2 Put the bananas into a mini food processor and add the coffee mixture and blend until smooth.

Nut butter

181 calories per serving

2 bananas, chopped and frozen until firm

2 tbsp nut butter

Put the bananas and nut butter into a mini food processor and blend until smooth.

Mixed fruits

102 calories per serving

2 bananas, chopped and frozen until firm

1 tsp vanilla extract

100g frozen summer fruits

Put the bananas, vanilla extract and frozen berries into a mini food processor and blend until smooth.

TOM'S TIP

For an extra boost of protein, add 2 tablespoons of unsweetened, unflavoured protein powder to the food processor and whizz with the other ingredients.

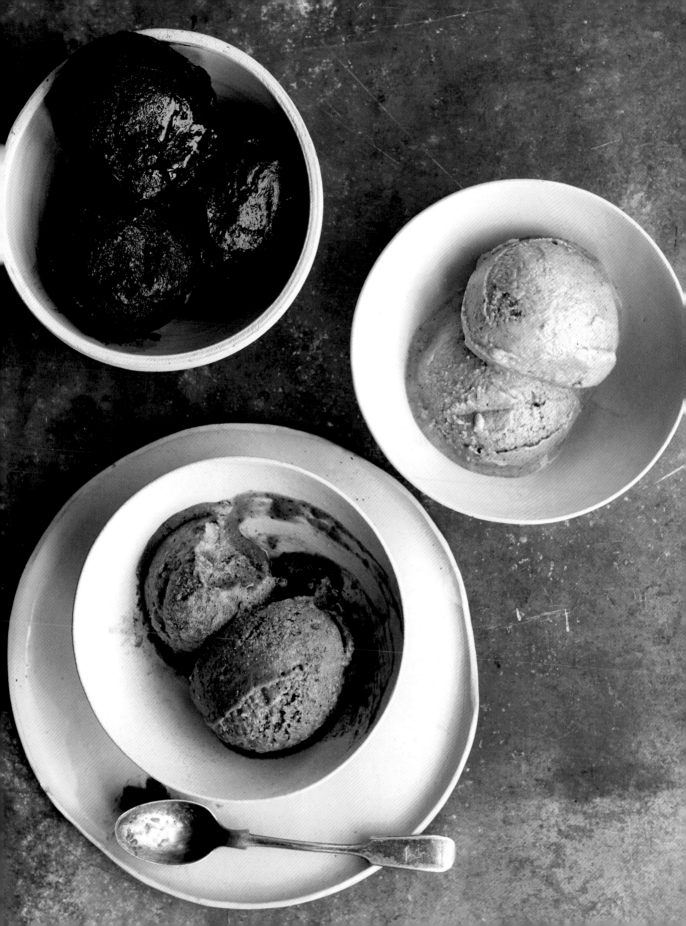

Millionaire shortbread puds

These are made in individual glasses and although they're less sweet than the traditional cake squares, they are still a fantastic treat.

SERVES 2
357 calories per serving

30g oats

15g whole almonds, roughly chopped

20g butter or coconut oil, melted

60g soft ready-to-eat dates

juice of 1 medium orange

30g dark chocolate (at least 85% cocoa solids)

1 Put the oats and almonds into a dry frying pan and toast for a few minutes until golden. Cool a little then tip into a mini blender and blitz until the mixture looks like fine crumbs. Remove the blade and stir in the melted butter or coconut oil, then divide evenly between two short glasses. Use the back of a teaspoon to press the mixture down until even. Transfer to the fridge to chill and set.

2 Put the dates into a small saucepan with the orange juice. Bring to the boil then turn the heat down to a simmer and cook for 6–7 minutes to soften.

3 Spoon the dates and any liquid in the pan into a mini blender and add 2 tablespoons of water. Blend until smooth then divide between the two glasses. Return to the fridge to chill.

4 Melt the chocolate in the microwave at the lowest power setting for 5–6 minutes, checking and stirring occasionally after every couple of minutes. Divide between the glasses and return to the fridge for 20–30 minutes to set.

Apple snow crumble

I've given this traditional recipe a twist and served it with a crunchy, quick-to-make crumble topping. Take care when baking the topping, as the edges will cook more quickly than the middle. Just don't spread it out too thinly or it may burn. Choose authentic Greek yoghurt, which is packed with protein and probiotics to give your immune system a boost!

SERVES 2
321 calories per serving

1 Bramley apple (about 300g), peeled, cored and chopped

1 tbsp maple syrup

75g Greek yoghurt

1 large egg white

For the crumble

2 tbsp regular oats

15g pecan nuts, finely chopped

10g butter, at room temperature

1 tbsp maple syrup

1 Preheat the oven to 200°C/180°C Fan/Gas 6.

2 Put the chopped apple into a saucepan and add the maple syrup and 2 tablespoons of water. Place over a low-medium heat and simmer for 5–6 minutes until the apple has softened and cooked through. Spoon into a bowl and mash until smooth.

3 Make the crumble by putting all the ingredients in a bowl and mixing until the butter is well incorporated. Spoon on to a baking tray into a small round circle – don't spread the mixture out too thinly or it will burn. Bake for 5–6 minutes until golden, watching it carefully. Leave to cool on the tray.

4 Fold the Greek yoghurt into the apple mixture. Whisk the egg white in a clean bowl until stiff peaks form – it'll take a couple of minutes if you're using a balloon whisk but shouldn't be too strenuous. Fold the beaten egg white into the apple mixture then divide between two bowls. Sprinkle the crumble evenly over the top and serve.

Peach & walnut split

This pudding is quick to rustle up and really filling, too. Make a speedy, creamy ice cream by mixing Greek yoghurt with honey and freezing in balls then sandwich between grilled peaches. Drizzle with melted chocolate for a touch of sweetness.

SERVES 2
194 calories per serving

2 heaped tbsp Greek yoghurt

1 tsp vanilla extract

2 tsp honey

2 peaches, halved and stoned

pinch of ground cinnamon

10g dark chocolate

10g white chocolate

4 walnuts, finely chopped

1 Mix the Greek yoghurt, vanilla extract and 1 teaspoon of the honey together then divide the mixture in two and spoon on to a plate, spaced apart. Roughly shape each portion into a round. Transfer to the freezer for 20–25 minutes until firm.

2 Preheat the grill and put the peaches, cut side up, on to a baking tray. Drizzle with the remaining honey and sprinkle over a little cinnamon. Grill for 7–8 minutes until golden.

3 Put each of the chocolates into separate small bowls and microwave at the lowest power setting for 2–3 minutes, stirring occasionally, until just melted.

4 Get out two plates and put a peach half on to each one. Spoon the frozen yoghurt in the middle and rest the other peach half on top of the yoghurt. Drizzle over the two chocolates and serve, scattered with the chopped walnuts.

I ALSO LOVE NECTARINES AND EVEN FRESH APRICOTS INSTEAD OF PEACHES. YOU'LL NEED 2-3 APRICOTS IN PLACE OF EACH PEACH

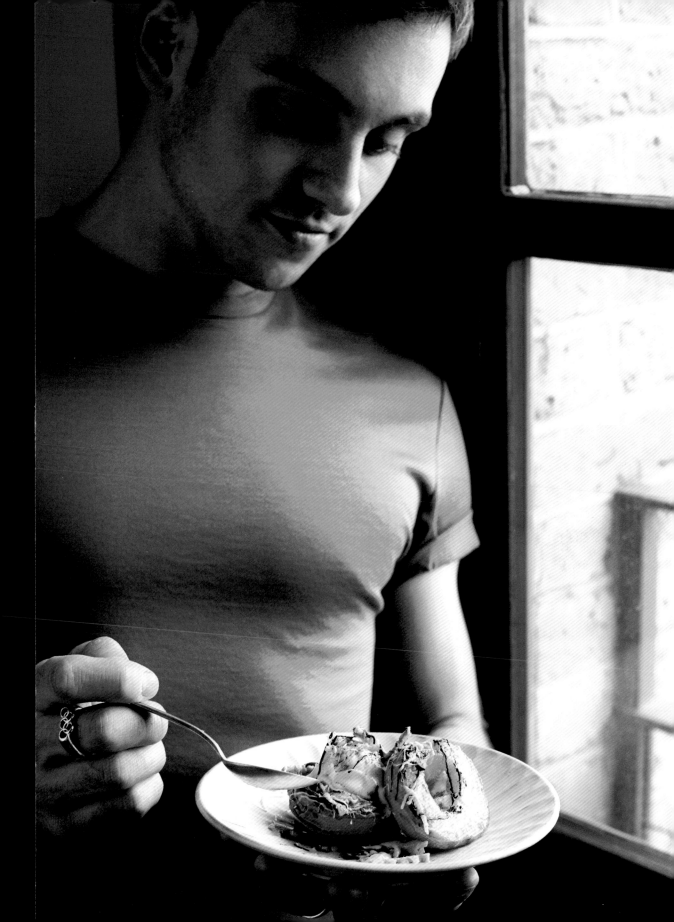

Tom & Lance's cupcake treats

These cakes are made from a very simple all-in-one mix, then half are flavoured with banana for me, and half with carrot for Lance. Instead of a gloopy icing, I've topped them with a thin layer of cream cheese – it's just enough to offset the sweetness of the cakes. The mix makes four cakes so freeze two for another time.

MAKES 4 CUPCAKES
318/328 calories per serving

For the basic mixture

1 large egg

65g butter, at room temperature

65g golden caster sugar

65g self-raising flour (or use half with wholemeal self-raising flour)

zest of 1 orange

1 tbsp freshly squeezed orange juice

For Tom's banana cupcakes

1/2 ripe banana (45g peeled weight), mashed

15g cream cheese

2 slices of banana

pinch of ground cinnamon

For Lance's carrot cupcakes

1/2 carrot (45g), grated

15g cream cheese

4 pecan nuts (8g)

pinch of ground cinnamon

1 Preheat the oven to 190°C/170°C Fan/Gas 5 and line a muffin tin with paper cases.

2 Crack the egg into a bowl then add the butter, sugar, flour, orange zest and orange juice. Use a hand-held electric whisk to beat everything together until smooth.

3 Spoon half into another bowl, then stir the mashed banana into one bowl of cake mix and the grated carrot into the other.

4 Divide the banana cake mix evenly between two muffin cases then do the same with the carrot cake mix. Bake for 25 minutes, or until a skewer inserted into the centre comes out clean. Lift out of the tin and cool on a wire rack.

5 Once cool spread the cream cheese evenly over the tops and decorate with the banana slices or pecan nuts. Finish with a sprinkle of cinnamon.

TOM'S TIP

To freeze any cakes that you're not eating straight away, wrap them without any topping in cling film and freeze for up to 3 months. To defrost, take out of the freezer and set aside on a plate for 1–2 hours until thoroughly defrosted.

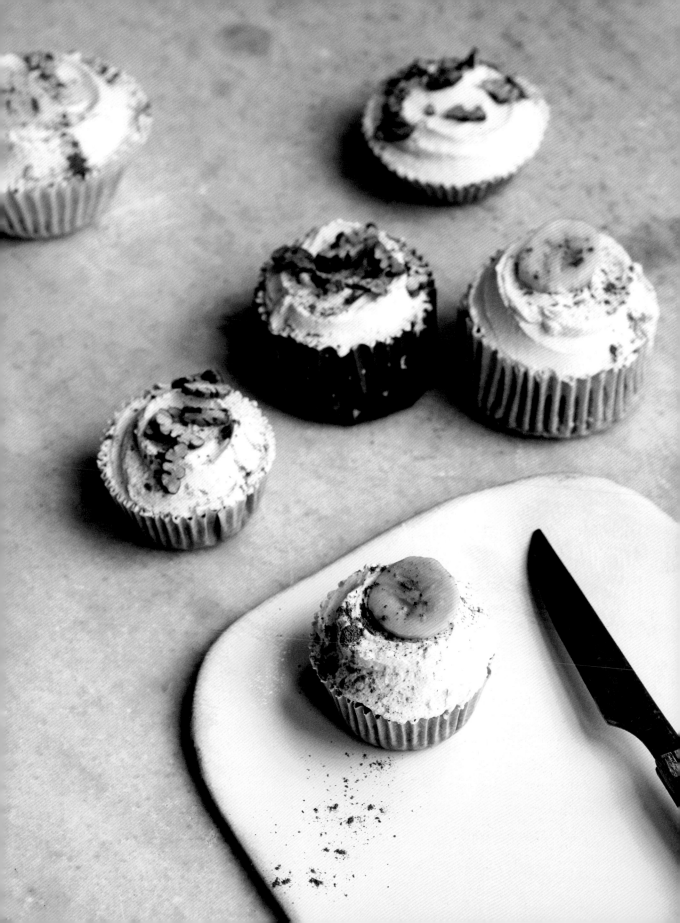

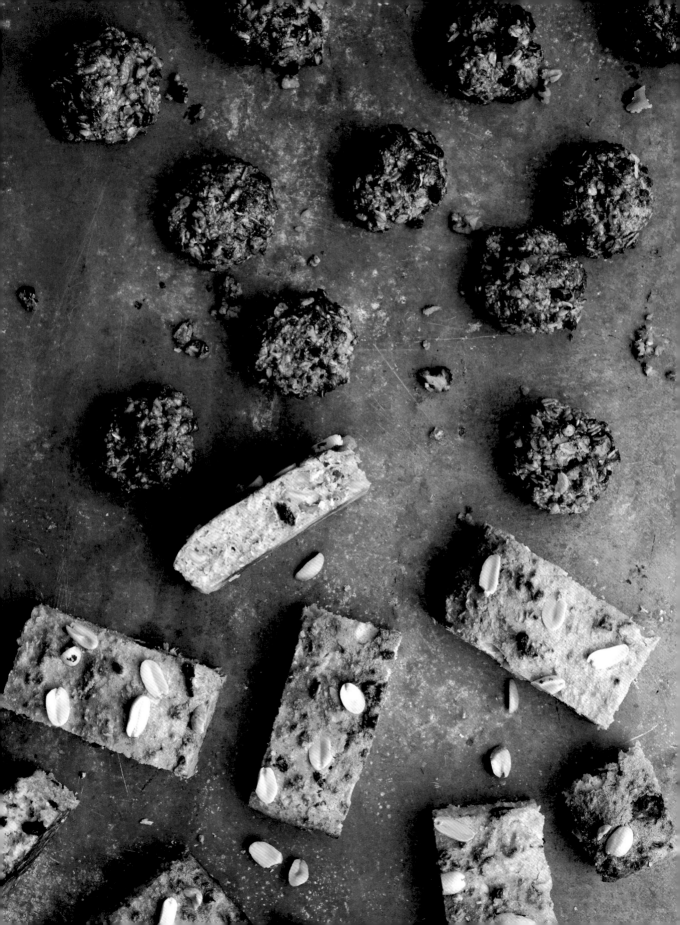

Pear & walnut oaties

These little bites are made from nuts, oil, pears, oats and spices. They're baked in the oven until firm and also contain a scoop of protein powder for an extra protein boost.

Makes 18 oaties
124 calories per serving

1 large pear (about 225g), peeled, cored
and chopped
30g unsweetened plain protein powder
1 tsp ground cinnamon or ginger
200g regular oats
100g walnuts, chopped
2¹/₂–3 tbsp sunflower oil or light olive oil
4 tbsp maple syrup

1 Preheat the oven to 200°C/180°C Fan/Gas 6 and line a large baking sheet with baking parchment.

2 Put the pear, protein powder, spice and half the oats into the bowl of a food processor and pulse briefly, just enough to roughly chop the pear and oats and combine the mixture. Spoon into a bowl and stir in the remaining oats, walnuts, sunflower oil and maple syrup. Mix everything together to make a rough dough.

3 Use a tablespoon measure to scoop up portions of the mixture. Roll each piece in the palm of your hand to make a ball then put on the lined baking sheet. Continue until you've rolled all the pieces to make 18 balls.

4 Bake in the oven for 18–20 minutes until golden all over, then leave to cool. Store in a sealable container for 4 days or freeze for up to one month.

Peanut & sultana protein bar

Here's a baked treat that also packs a protein punch. I've used healthy oats instead of flour and supplemented them with protein powder. They keep in a sealed container for 4 days or can be frozen for up to one month.

Makes 12 bars
249 calories per serving

100g unsalted peanuts
3 medium eggs
75g honey
1 ripe banana (about 125g peeled weight), mashed
100g unsweetened plain protein powder
100g oats
75g butter, melted and cooled
50g desiccated coconut
75g sultanas
good pinch of salt

1 Preheat the oven to 200°C/180°C Fan/Gas 6 and line a 20cm square tin with baking parchment.

2 Tip the peanuts on to a baking sheet and roast in the oven for 5 minutes until just golden. Don't let them get too dark or they'll taste bitter and burnt. Tip on to a board and roughly chop then set aside.

3 Beat the eggs and honey together in a large bowl until the eggs have mixed into the honey and the mixture looks frothy. Fold in the mashed banana, protein powder, oats, melted butter, desiccated coconut, sultanas and salt, along with 150ml water. Stir to mix everything together well.

4 Spoon the mixture into the tin and level it out so it's even on top then bake for 20–25 minutes, or until golden brown on top and firm.

Nutritional Information

To make it easy for you to see the nutritional values of the recipes, I've provided a breakdown for each one, giving the calories and the amount in grams of protein, carbohydrate, sugar, fat, saturated fat, fibre and salt. My recipes will show that you don't need to indulge in high-calorie foods to enjoy mouth-watering meals! The sugar content given includes the natural sugars in foods such as milk and fruit as well as free sugars – the sugar added to food. The calculations don't include any optional ingredients.

Figures below are per serving, unless otherwise specified. I also list how much each recipe contributes to your recommended '5 a day' fruit and veggie intake. One portion is about 80 grams and five portions of fruit and veg is the minimum amount – research now shows that 10 portions will decrease the risk of disease – so the more the better!

For someone eating 2,000 calories a day, the suggested level of intake of nutrients is as follows:

Protein 45g

Carbs 270g

Sugar 90g

Fat 70g

Saturated fat 20g

Fibre 30g

Salt 6g

BREAKFASTS

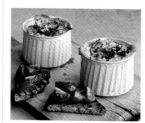

Smoky beans in a bun (page 79)

2 of your 5 a day
Kcals: 231
Protein (g) 11
Carbs (g) 31
Sugar (g) 4
Fat (g) 5
Sat fat (g) 1
Fibre (g) 5
Salt (g) 0.5

Smoked salmon & courgette breakfast pots (page 80)

1 of your 5 a day
Kcals: 318
Protein (g) 30
Carbs (g) 15
Sugar (g) 4
Fat (g) 14
Sat fat (g) 4
Fibre (g) 4
Salt (g) 2.5

Tom's extra special slow-cooked eggs (page 82)

Kcals: 394
Protein (g) 28
Carbs (g) 20
Sugar (g) 2
Fat (g) 23
Sat fat (g) 9
Fibre (g) 1
Salt (g) 2

Poached egg & avocado on toasted pitta (page 84)

1 of your 5 a day
Kcals: 360
Protein (g) 18.5
Carbs (g) 30
Sugar (g) 4.5
Fat (g) 17
Sat fat (g) 4.5
Fibre (g) 7
Salt (g) 1.2

Bacon & chestnut mushrooms on toast (page 85)

1 of your 5 a day
Kcals: 358
Protein (g) 17
Carbs (g) 23
Sugar (g) 3
Fat (g) 20
Sat fat (g) 4
Fibre (g) 5
Salt (g) 2.2

The ultimate sausage sandwich (page 86)

1 of your 5 a day
Kcals: 275
Protein (g) 21
Carbs (g) 24
Sugar (g) 4
Fat (g) 9
Sat fat (g) 3.5
Fibre (g) 3.5
Salt (g) 2

Sweetcorn pancakes (page 88)

2 of your 5 a day
Kcals: 266
Protein (g) 16
Carbs (g) 10
Sugar (g) 5
Fat (g) 18
Sat fat (g) 3
Fibre (g) 2.5
Salt (g) 1.2

Spiced apricot & almond porridge (page 90)

Kcals: 324
Protein (g) 8
Carbs (g) 28
Sugar (g) 7.5
Fat (g) 18
Sat fat (g) 8
Fibre (g) 4.4
Salt (g) trace

Raspberry & fig Bircher muesli (page 91)

1 of your 5 a day
Kcals: 450
Protein (g) 15
Carbs (g) 42
Sugar (g) 24
Fat (g) 23
Sat fat (g) 9
Fibre (g) 8
Salt (g) 0.3

Cottage cheese pots (page 92)

1 of your 5 a day
Kcals: 290
Protein (g) 14
Carbs (g) 8
Sugar (g) 5
Fat (g) 22
Sat fat (g) 4
Fibre (g) 4
Salt (g) 0.5

LIGHT LUNCHES & SALADS

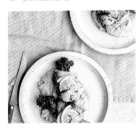

Pea & ham soup (page 95)

2 of your 5 a day

Kcals: 330
Protein (g) 25
Carbs (g) 28
Sugar (g) 3.5
Fat (g) 11
Sat fat (g) 4
Fibre (g) 7
Salt (g) 3

Thai-style squash & noodle soup (page 96)

3 of your 5 a day

Kcals: 474
Protein (g) 22
Carbs (g) 68
Sugar (g) 13
Fat (g) 11
Sat fat (g) 4
Fibre (g) 9
Salt (g) 0.7

Tartine for vegans (page 99)

1 of your 5 a day

Kcals: 264
Protein (g) 8
Carbs (g) 27
Sugar (g) 13
Fat (g) 11.5
Sat fat (g) 1.5
Fibre (g) 8
Salt (g) 0.8

Tartine for vegetarians (page 99)

Kcals: 300
Protein (g) 13
Carbs (g) 21
Sugar (g) 4
Fat (g) 18
Sat fat (g) 9
Fibre (g) 3
Salt (g) 2

Tartine for fish-lovers (page 99)

Kcals: 303
Protein (g) 28
Carbs (g) 19
Sugar (g) 1.5
Fat (g) 12
Sat fat (g) 3
Fibre (g) 3.5
Salt (g) 1.5

Tartine for meat-lovers (page 99)

1 of your 5 a day

Kcals: 237
Protein (g) 20
Carbs (g) 21
Sugar (g) 4
Fat (g) 7
Sat fat (g) 2
Fibre (g) 4.5
Salt (g) 1

Warm salmon salad (page 100)

2 of your 5 a day

Kcals: 390
Protein (g) 32
Carbs (g) 19
Sugar (g) 7
Fat (g) 19
Sat fat (g) 3
Fibre (g) 10
Salt (g) 1.2

Autumn salad (page 101)

3 of your 5 a day

Kcals: 460
Protein (g) 12
Carbs (g) 36
Sugar (g) 22
Fat (g) 26
Sat fat (g) 3.5
Fibre (g) 15
Salt (g) trace

Crayfish cocktail with a Mexican twist (page 102)

1 of your 5 a day

Kcals: 152
Protein (g) 11
Carbs (g) 4
Sugar (g) 3
Fat (g) 10
Sat fat (g) 2
Fibre (g) 3.5
Salt (g) 0.3

Italian salad (page 104)

3 of your 5 a day

Kcals: 561
Protein (g) 25
Carbs (g) 35
Sugar (g) 6
Fat (g) 34
Sat fat (g) 11
Fibre (g) 8
Salt (g) 1.2

Mediterranean mezze salad (page 106)

2 of your 5 a day

Kcals: 485
Protein (g) 18
Carbs (g) 41
Sugar (g) 5
Fat (g) 25
Sat fat (g) 2
Fibre (g) 13
Salt (g) 0.9

Warm quinoa salad with kale crisps (page 107)

2 of your 5 a day

Kcals: 400
Protein (g) 21
Carbs (g) 43
Sugar (g) 12
Fat (g) 14
Sat fat (g) 2.5
Fibre (g) 14
Salt (g) 0.7

Tom's rainbow salad (page 108)

4 of your 5 a day

Kcals: 445
Protein (g) 19
Carbs (g) 17
Sugar (g) 15
Fat (g) 32
Sat fat (g) 8.5
Fibre (g) 8
Salt (g) 0.8

Tom's Buddha bowl (page 110)

3 of your 5 a day

Kcals: 367
Protein (g) 22
Carbs (g) 17
Sugar (g) 8
Fat (g) 20
Sat fat (g) 3
Fibre (g) 14
Salt (g) 0.1

Chicken satay with Asian slaw (page 112)

2 of your 5 a day

Kcals: 470
Protein (g) 45
Carbs (g) 13
Sugar (g) 11
Fat (g) 24
Sat fat (g) 4
Fibre (g) 10
Salt (g) 1.8

READY IN 15

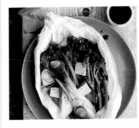

Pea & tomato omelette with feta (page 115)

2 of your 5 a day

Kcals: 337
Protein (g) 25
Carbs (g) 11
Sugar (g) 5
Fat (g) 20
Sat fat (g) 9.5
Fibre (g) 5
Salt (g) 1.1

Hot chilli prawns with crisp salad (page 116)

4 of your 5 a day

Kcals: 336
Protein (g) 39
Carbs (g) 22
Sugar (g) 15
Fat (g) 8
Sat fat (g) 1.5
Fibre (g) 8
Salt (g) 1.7

Quick healthy fried eggs (page 118)

3 of your 5 a day

Kcals: 333
Protein (g) 24
Carbs (g) 15
Sugar (g) 13
Fat (g) 18
Sat fat (g) 8
Fibre (g) 6.5
Salt (g) 0.7

Quick lemon chicken with steamed veg (page 120)

3 of your 5 a day

Kcals: 302
Protein (g) 42
Carbs (g) 10
Sugar (g) 8
Fat (g) 9
Sat fat (g) 1.5
Fibre (g) 7.5
Salt (g) 0.3

Speedy tofu pasta (page 121)

1 of your 5 a day

Kcals: 680
Protein (g) 33
Carbs (g) 76
Sugar (g) 5
Fat (g) 24
Sat fat (g) 3
Fibre (g) 12
Salt (g) 0.2

Steamed tofu parcel (page 122)

3 of your 5 a day

Kcals: 194
Protein (g) 15
Carbs (g) 17
Sugar (g) 15
Fat (g) 6
Sat fat (g) 1
Fibre (g) 8
Salt (g) 1.6

Healthy steamed salmon (page 124)

1 of your 5 a day

Kcals: 526
Protein (g) 40
Carbs (g) 12
Sugar (g) 4.5
Fat (g) 33.5
Sat fat (g) 7
Fibre (g) 8.5
Salt (g) 0.2

SUPPERS

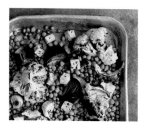

Tom's pesto pasta (page 127)

2 of your 5 a day
Kcals: 580
Protein (g) 19
Carbs (g) 66
Sugar (g) 6
Fat (g) 24
Sat fat (g) 5
Fibre (g) 10
Salt (g) 0.2

Chicken & tenderstem broccoli wraps (page 128)

2 of your 5 a day
Kcals: 550
Protein (g) 54
Carbs (g) 24
Sugar (g) 2
Fat (g) 23.5
Sat fat (g) 7.5
Fibre (g) 13
Salt (g) 2

Baked peppers (page 130)

4 of your 5 a day
Kcals: 408
Protein (g) 15
Carbs (g) 52
Sugar (g) 16
Fat (g) 10.5
Sat fat (g) 1.5
Fibre (g) 22
Salt (g) 0.5

Parmesan cod with quick Mediterranean vegetables (page 131)

4 of your 5 a day
Kcals: 326
Protein (g) 33
Carbs (g) 10
Sugar (g) 10
Fat (g) 16
Sat fat (g) 4
Fibre (g) 7
Salt (g) 0.6

Tuna with mango & lime (page 132)

2 of your 5 a day
Kcals: 500
Protein (g) 48
Carbs (g) 58
Sugar (g) 13
Fat (g) 7
Sat fat (g) 1.5
Fibre (g) 6.5
Salt (g) 0.4

Pan-fried mackerel with new potato salad (page 134)

2 of your 5 a day
Kcals: 606
Protein (g) 41
Carbs (g) 32
Sugar (g) 6
Fat (g) 32
Sat fat (g) 7.5
Fibre (g) 12.5
Salt (g) 0.6

Salmon poké bowl (page 136)

2 of your 5 a day
Kcals: 714
Protein (g) 44
Carbs (g) 49
Sugar (g) 4
Fat (g) 36
Sat fat (g) 6.5
Fibre (g) 8
Salt (g) 1

Sweet potato pan-fry with cheesy steak (page 138)

3 of your 5 a day
Kcals: 433
Protein (g) 35
Carbs (g) 27
Sugar (g) 13
Fat (g) 19
Sat fat (g) 5
Fibre (g) 9
Salt (g) 0.4

Chicken meatballs with orzo, parsley & lemon (page 140)

3 of your 5 a day
Kcals: 592
Protein (g) 63
Carbs (g) 55
Sugar (g) 16
Fat (g) 11
Sat fat (g) 2.5
Fibre (g) 9.5
Salt (g) 1

Lean lamb cutlets with beans (page 142)

2 of your 5 a day
Kcals: 350
Protein (g) 32
Carbs (g) 16.5
Sugar (g) 2.5
Fat (g) 15.5
Sat fat (g) 4.5
Fibre (g) 11
Salt (g) 0.22

Teriyaki noodles with marinated tofu (page 143)

3 of your 5 a day
Kcals: 626
Protein (g) 32
Carbs (g) 62
Sugar (g) 19
Fat (g) 25
Sat fat (g) 8.5
Fibre (g) 10
Salt (g) 1.9

Spicy vegetable bean stew with giant croutons (page 144)

3 of your 5 a day
Kcals: 373
Protein (g) 14
Carbs (g) 37
Sugar (g) 10
Fat (g) 16
Sat fat (g) 5
Fibre (g) 12
Salt (g) 1

Quick-roast cauli with chickpeas & Indian spices (page 146)

4 of your 5 a day
Kcals: 500
Protein (g) 26
Carbs (g) 50
Sugar (g) 20
Fat (g) 18
Sat fat (g) 3
Fibre (g) 17
Salt (g) 5

WEEKEND FEASTS

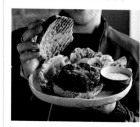

Chickpea korma (page 149)

2 of your 5 a day
Kcals: 738
Protein (g) 28
Carbs (g) 74
Sugar (g) 9
Fat (g) 33
Sat fat (g) 9
Fibre (g) 15
Salt (g) 0.65

One-pot gammon with roots (page 150)

3 of your 5 a day
Kcals: 382
Protein (g) 32
Carbs (g) 23
Sugar (g) 11
Fat (g) 16
Sat fat (g) 6
Fibre (g) 10
Salt (g) 3.5

One-pot sort of Sunday roast for two (page 152)

5 of your 5 a day
Kcals: 511
Protein (g) 36
Carbs (g) 45
Sugar (g) 24
Fat (g) 15
Sat fat (g) 5
Fibre (g) 20
Salt (g) 1.2

Veggie Bolognese (page 153)

1 of your 5 a day
Kcals: 447
Protein (g) 24
Carbs (g) 68
Sugar (g) 6
Fat (g) 6
Sat fat (g) 2
Fibre (g) 11
Salt (g) 1.5

Giant spring rolls with tofu & sesame (page 154)

1 of your 5 a day
Kcals: 200
Protein (g) 7.5
Carbs (g) 27
Sugar (g) 8
Fat (g) 6
Sat fat (g) 1.5
Fibre (g) 5
Salt (g) 1.2

Roast chicken with vegetable bake (page 156)

1 of your 5 a day
Kcals: 470
Protein (g) 43
Carbs (g) 10
Sugar (g) 8
Fat (g) 21
Sat fat (g) 6
Fibre (g) 4
Salt (g) 0.5

Tom's Olympic burger (page 160)

Kcals: 792
Protein (g) 60
Carbs (g) 58
Sugar (g) 8.5
Fat (g) 34
Sat fat (g) 13
Fibre (g) 9
Salt (g) 2.4

Cheat's turkey mole (page 162)

2 of your 5 a day

Kcals: 644
Protein (g) 51
Carbs (g) 69
Sugar (g) 13.5
Fat (g) 15.5
Sat fat (g) 4
Fibre (g) 11
Salt (g) 1

Crunchy chicken & sweet potato chips (page 164)

2 of your 5 a day

Kcals: 644
Protein (g) 51
Carbs (g) 69
Sugar (g) 13.5
Fat (g) 15.5
Sat fat (g) 4
Fibre (g) 11
Salt (g) 1

Aubergine & sweet potato cake (page 166)

3 of your 5 a day

Kcals: 238
Protein (g) 9
Carbs (g) 24
Sugar (g) 10
Fat (g) 10
Sat fat (g) 3.5
Fibre (g) 7
Salt (g) 0.7

Sausage & smash (page 168)

1 of your 5 a day

Kcals: 436
Protein (g) 37
Carbs (g) 45
Sugar (g) 12
Fat (g) 10
Sat fat (g) 3
Fibre (g) 9
Salt (g) 0.3

My all-the-veg pasta bake (page 170)

3 of your 5 a day

Kcals: 472
Protein (g) 23
Carbs (g) 52
Sugar (g) 15
Fat (g) 18
Sat fat (g) 9.5
Fibre (g) 7.5
Salt (g) 1.6

Braised beef with beans & roasted broccoli (page 171)

2 of your 5 a day

Kcals: 473
Protein (g) 59
Carbs (g) 21
Sugar (g) 5
Fat (g) 15
Sat fat (g) 4
Fibre (g) 10
Salt (g) 1.4

DESSERTS & DRINKS

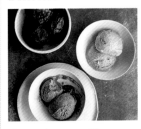

The anytime smoothie (page 173)

Kcals: 249
Protein (g) 11
Carbs (g) 29
Sugar (g) 21
Fat (g) 9
Sat fat (g) 1
Fibre (g) 5.5
Salt (g) 0.05

Virgin orange mojito (page 173)

1 of your 5 a day

Kcals: 50
Protein (g) 1
Carbs (g) 11.5
Sugar (g) 11.5
Fat (g) 0
Sat fat (g) 0
Fibre (g) 0
Salt (g) 0

Piña colada smoothie (page 173)

1 of your 5 a day

Kcals: 160
Protein (g) 4
Carbs (g) 16
Sugar (g) 16
Fat (g) 8
Sat fat (g) 6
Fibre (g) 4
Salt (g) 0.1

Berry parcels with a chocolate sauce (page 174)

Kcals: 167
Protein (g) 2
Carbs (g) 26
Sugar (g) 15
Fat (g) 6
Sat fat (g) 2
Fibre (g) 2
Salt (g) 0.1

Tom's dead easy banana ice cream – cinnamon (page 176)

1 of your 5 a day

Kcals: 86
Protein (g) 1
Carbs (g) 19
Sugar (g) 17
Fat (g) 0
Sat fat (g) 0
Fibre (g) 1.5
Salt (g) 0

Tom's dead easy banana ice cream – nut butter (page 176)

1 of your 5 a day

Kcals: 181
Protein (g) 5
Carbs (g) 21
Sugar (g) 18
Fat (g) 8
Sat fat (g) 2
Fibre (g) 2.5
Salt (g) 0.1

Tom's dead easy banana ice cream – mixed fruits (page 176)

1 of your 5 a day

Kcals: 102
Protein (g) 1.5
Carbs (g) 21.5
Sugar (g) 19.5
Fat (g) 0
Sat fat (g) 0
Fibre (g) 3
Salt (g) 0

Millionaire shortbread puds (page 178)

Kcals: 357
Protein (g) 5
Carbs (g) 42
Sugar (g) 30
Fat (g) 18
Sat fat (g) 8
Fibre (g) 4
Salt (g) 0.2

Apple snow crumble (page 179)

1 of your 5 a day

Kcals: 321
Protein (g) 7
Carbs (g) 38
Sugar (g) 26
Fat (g) 15
Sat fat (g) 6
Fibre (g) 4
Salt (g) 0.2

Peach & walnut split (page 180)

1 of your 5 a day

Kcals: 194
Protein (g) 4
Carbs (g) 24
Sugar (g) 24
Fat (g) 8.5
Sat fat (g) 4
Fibre (g) 3.5
Salt (g) 0

Tom's banana cupcakes (page 182)

Kcals: 318
Protein (g) 4.5
Carbs (g) 36
Sugar (g) 23
Fat (g) 17
Sat fat (g) 10
Fibre (g) 1
Salt (g) 0.6

Lance's carrot cupcakes (page 182)

Kcals: 328
Protein (g) 5
Carbs (g) 32
Sugar (g) 19
Fat (g) 20
Sat fat (g) 10
Fibre (g) 2
Salt (g) 0.6

Pear & walnut oaties (page 184)

Kcals: 124
Protein (g) 3.5
Carbs (g) 12
Sugar (g) 5
Fat (g) 6.5
Sat fat (g) 0.8
Fibre (g) 1.5
Salt (g) 0

Peanut & sultana protein bar (page 184)

Kcals: 249
Protein (g) 12.5
Carbs (g) 18
Sugar (g) 12
Fat (g) 14
Sat fat (g) 7
Fibre (g) 2
Salt (g) 0.3

6.00

7.00

8.00

9.00

10.00

11.00

12.00

13.00

14.00

15.00 ◀ **3.00** **P.M.**

16.00

17.00

18.00

19.00

20.00

21.00

22.00

23.00

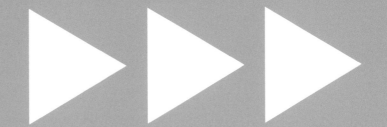

HABIT 5
STRESS & RESILIENCE

Since the age of about seven or eight, I have always kept a diary, where I record what I have been doing for my training and why. Some days I write more than on others. As well as recording events in your life, in a journal you also record your emotions and feelings around those events so you can gain clarity and make positive changes. Some of the most influential people in history are said to have kept journals: Albert Einstein, Marie Curie, Charles Darwin, Isaac Newton and Leonardo di Vinci all wrote down their daily thoughts and ideas.

There is a growing body of research and mounting evidence to show that keeping a journal has a positive impact on mental and emotional well-being. Some experts believe that writing about stressful events can help us process and come to terms with them, reducing the impact on our physical health. Once we release the force of emotions in this way, we can feel calmer and more peaceful. Research for the University of Arizona found that keeping a journal after going through a divorce helped people to not only make sense of the experience on an emotional level and move forward but they also showed higher heart rate variability and a lower heart rate, associated with improved physical health.

When we write a journal, we activate the left sides of our brains, which are more analytical and rational. It allows us to understand ourselves and the people around us better. Do you ever feel anxious, stressed or angry about something but are not sure why? Taking time out to write down what you feel might help you understand yourself and your emotions more clearly. This allows us to be more self-aware and feel calmer. However, when we use our left brains to solve problems, it doesn't always resolve the issue. If we also tap into our intuitive right brain when writing, we can brainstorm new ideas and find unexpected solutions to problems we are tackling.

Regular journalling can serve as a reminder of the mistakes we have made, our proudest moments and achievements and the moments we want to remember. This can come in handy when we are worried or feeling down and can be used as a tool to make us feel better, to see how we tackled a similar problem last time or to think about how we could approach it differently. Often, our fears about something are far worse than the situation itself and by writing them down, it helps us to see things more clearly because we become more conscious of the way we react to stressful events. We can see patterns in our behaviour or actions that can allow us to move forward in a positive way.

I journal my stresses and anxieties around relationships that I have within my sport. Sometimes it can be really useful to write down the way you feel about someone in a certain situation, to help you see it clearly and understand how you can tackle it. I also find it useful for detailing my thoughts around stressful situations within diving. After 2012, when I had to do a 're-dive' on my back twisting dive, I was so terrified about ever doing it again that it started to weigh on my everyday life. I was frightened of doing anything different or outside of my routine for fear that something would go wrong. So I started to write down these feelings and thinking about what was making me feel that way. We then started to investigate the dive itself and made changes, which meant inventing a completely new dive! My coach came into training one day with a video of someone performing a forward three-and-a-half somersaults with one twist on a Russian swing in a circus. So that's what we did. We took a circus trick and turned it into an Olympic dive!

Whether you use a paper notebook or one of the many journalling and diary apps on your phone or computer, journalling can help you to understand what makes you feel happy, confident and inspired. It is also a great way to build better habits because it forces us to be aware of our actions and behaviour. In this way, we are more likely to achieve our goals.

IF YOU DO ONE THING ...
Keep a learning journal documenting how you've approached and dealt with daily challenges. This will become an invaluable reference that will help you realise that day-to-day fears often aren't grounded in reality, and that you're a lot stronger and more resourceful than you think.

Healthy ways to calm anxiety

Feeling anxious is never a pleasant experience; from a racing heart, to sweating palms and feeling sick, stress has a horrible way of affecting our bodies and minds. Here are a few ways to calm yourself down when you are feeling anxious.

Reframe your thoughts
The physical symptoms of stress and anxiety are very similar to those of excitement. When these symptoms start, try to tell yourself that it is just the effects of adrenalin and it will pass. By reframing and controlling your thoughts in this way, you will be able to cope better with the situation.

Postpone it
If something – or a series of things – is worrying you, allocate some time in your diary at a later time or date to think about them. Chances are that by the time that moment comes round, the worry will have lessened. Allow yourself ten minutes to dwell on it: think of possible outcomes for the scenario, think of some actions and then move on.

Use a calming visualisation
When you are feeling stressed, close your eyes and picture yourself somewhere calm, in a place that makes you happy. This could be on the beach, by a river or in a favourite park. Think about the different things you can see, hear and touch. If your mind wanders, bring yourself back to the scene.

Eat well
When we are stressed and anxious, it can throw our bodies out of sync and we may lose our appetites or crave certain foods. It is important to give our bodies the support they need by eating foods high in vitamin B and omega-3 fatty acids, which are both linked to good mental health.

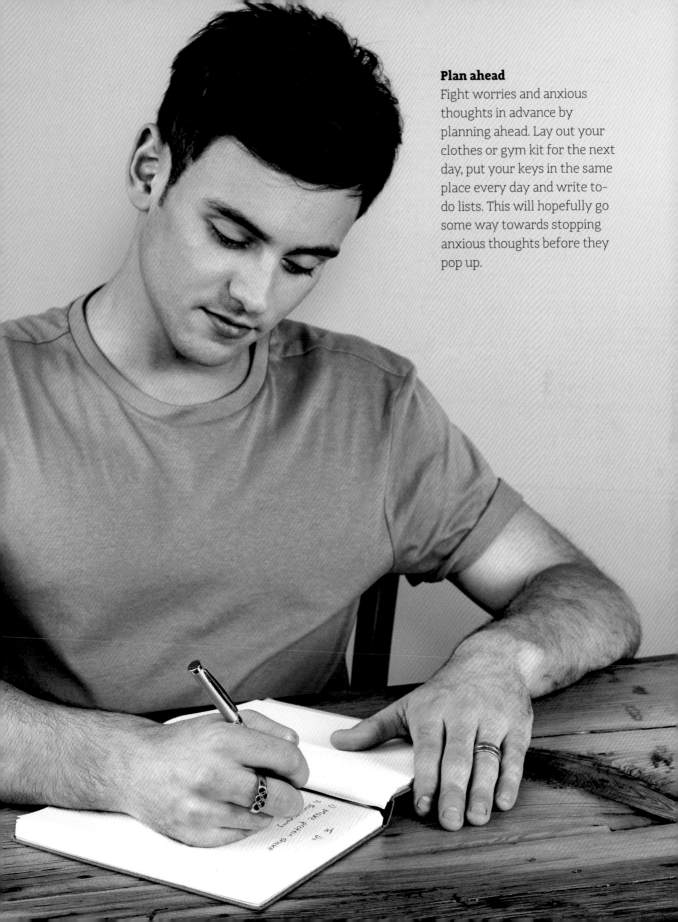

Plan ahead
Fight worries and anxious thoughts in advance by planning ahead. Lay out your clothes or gym kit for the next day, put your keys in the same place every day and write to-do lists. This will hopefully go some way towards stopping anxious thoughts before they pop up.

Top ways to foster resilience and stay mentally robust

Resilience has been defined as the ability to bounce back in times of adversity – basically not losing your cool when times are tough. It's not about avoiding stress; instead it's about facing the difficult times and learning from them. Research has shown that while some people are naturally more resilient than others, these types of behaviours can be learned and cultivated. Here are just a few ideas.

Create your own definition of success

Resilient people do not compare themselves with others. By working towards our own definition of success and trying to be the best we can, no one else matters. Everyone's journey is unique. In the world of sport, this is hard because we are constantly compared against one another. In sports like tennis, paying close attention to what competitors do is vital to success but in an individual sport, even if we watch and try to mimic what other people do, that might not work best for our bodies. The same applies to every area of life, so only by being the best we can are we doing ourselves justice. Our differences are what shape our individual lives.

Welcome change

Most of us fear change, simply because it is unknown. Change happens for a reason, so try to look at it as an opportunity. So, if a relationship ends, this gives you the chance to focus on or prioritise yourself, or if your company downsizes, this could be the chance for you to pursue your dream job.

Be realistic

It is important to try not to see situations in black and white. Don't assume that if something is not a complete success, it is therefore a failure. If you were a friend looking in on the situation, what would you say? Having a more optimistic outlook enables you to see that good things will happen in your life. After the 2016 Olympics, I felt heartbroken. However, I have managed to look back and see that it was a success because I won a bronze medal. If someone had told me before the event that I would come home with an Olympic bronze medal, I would have been over the moon, so over time, I have taken the positives from that experience away with me.

Use your mental energy wisely

When time and energy are limited, there is no point worrying about things that are beyond your control or overthinking the past, which cannot be changed. Empower yourself to use your mental energy to tune into being truly present in the moment and to focus on things you can change.

Become physically stronger

It might seem counter-intuitive but it is possible to become mentally tougher if you are physically stronger. Part of being resilient is that you feel you have control over your responses to difficult situations and if you are out of shape, this can lead you to feel less in control.

Stay social

Research has shown that the impact of relationships on all areas of our well-being is huge. When times are tough, it can feel like you just want to be alone and deal with it by yourself but one of the best things you can do is spend time with friends and family. By talking through problems, you can help solve them more quickly.

5 ways to bounce back from mistakes as a more confident person

1

Focus on working hard:
Rather than thinking about where you went wrong, focus your attention on ways of becoming better. Accomplishments lead to increased confidence and working hard will help you achieve your goals.

2

Learn positive reframing:
Whatever has happened, put it into perspective and focus on what went right rather than what didn't. Look at the situation from the outside and ask a friend for their opinion.

ALWAYS OWN YOUR MISTAKES AND ACCEPT THE CONSEQUENCES; ONLY THEN WILL YOU BE ABLE TO MOVE ON

People often ask me how I bounce back from competitions where I feel disappointed. Sometimes it's not easy but I always manage to look forward. Whether you have messed up in an exam or interview, made a personal error or another mistake, here are some ideas about how you can do the same.

3

Take a break: It is really important to take some time out after big setbacks. I always try to take some time off after major competitions, even if it is just a few days, whether I have done well or not. I spend time with Lance, my family and my close friends and remember what truly matters in life! You have to give your brain a chance to recover after a stressful situation, not just your body. Recovery in all areas of your life is key to well-being.

4

Try not to beat yourself up: Research at the University of Berkeley in California shows that the ability to show self-compassion is not only a key driver of success but leads to less anxiety and conflict. By going over past mistakes you only serve to dent your confidence even more. Understand that one mistake does not define you.

5

Don't shrink your goals: Do not let negative emotions stop you from putting yourself back out there and trying again. Always set the bar high and aim for success. Real failure is when you do not try.

6.00

7.00

8.00

9.00

10.00

11.00

12.00

13.00

14.00

15.00

16.00

17.00

18.00

19.00

20.00 ◄ **8.00** P.M.

21.00

22.00

23.00

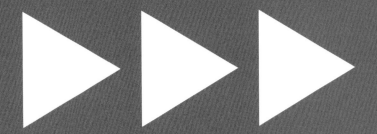

HABIT 6
DIGITAL DETOX

Tips for a total digital detox

Our lives are full of screens; we wake up to them, carry them around in our pockets all day and come home to them. Screens and social media allow creativity, enjoyment and connectivity but it is important to take time out every now and then. Here's how to make your digital detox a success.

Give yourself an allowance

Establish a maximum amount of time you can use your devices per day. By restricting time – rather than completely banning it – you are more likely to stick to it.

Go slowly

If you are very reliant on technology, start by setting small time limits each day, then increase the limits over time. This will help to create new habits and make your detox easier to stick to.

Change one habit at a time

Start by banning phones at the table, then from the bedroom, then allow yourself to check your email every two hours and so on. Remove your dependencies one at a time for lasting results.

Tell everyone what you are doing

The more people you tell about your digital detox, the more likely you are to stick to it.

Don't use your smartphone as an alarm clock

By using a normal alarm clock to wake up in the morning, you will avoid the temptation to browse Facebook, Instagram or Snapchat just before you go to bed, or the moment you open your eyes! If you must use your phone, switch it to night or aeroplane mode.

Take emails completely off your phone

Instant email response is increasingly seen as the norm but it adds to our stress levels at home and at work because we feel we should respond instantly to each important message we receive. Limit your ability to check and respond to emails by doing it once or twice a day via your desktop.

Compliment people in real life

How many times today have you 'liked' something on social media? Get used to complimenting people face-to-face.

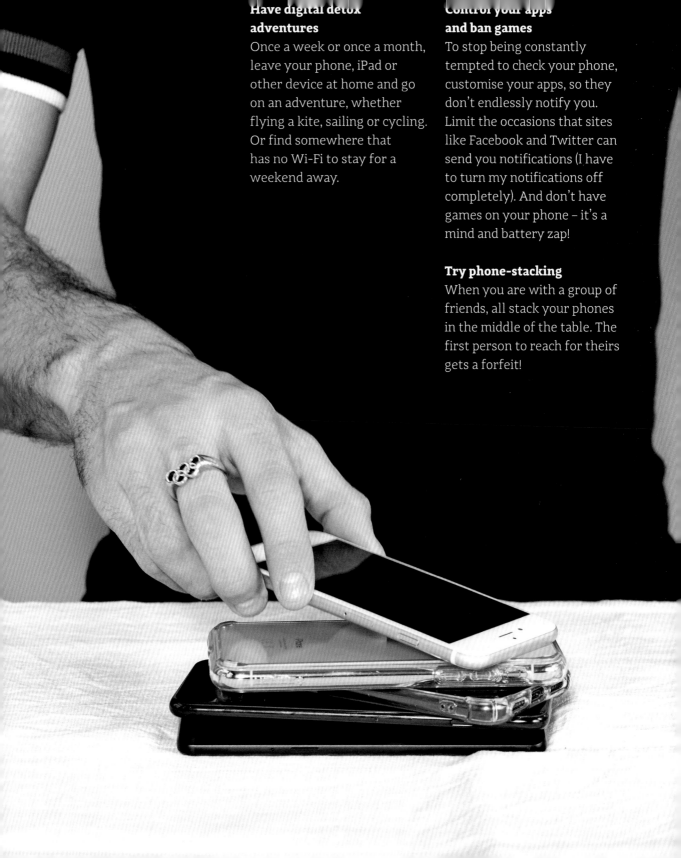

Have digital detox adventures

Once a week or once a month, leave your phone, iPad or other device at home and go on an adventure, whether flying a kite, sailing or cycling. Or find somewhere that has no Wi-Fi to stay for a weekend away.

Control your apps and ban games

To stop being constantly tempted to check your phone, customise your apps, so they don't endlessly notify you. Limit the occasions that sites like Facebook and Twitter can send you notifications (I have to turn my notifications off completely). And don't have games on your phone – it's a mind and battery zap!

Try phone-stacking

When you are with a group of friends, all stack your phones in the middle of the table. The first person to reach for theirs gets a forfeit!

How to use social media to inspire yourself

We all know that browsing social media can be a big drain on our time. But how can we use it as a tool rather than a distraction? So that rather than simply entertaining us, it inspires and motivates. Here are some ideas.

Unfriend and unfollow

There is a lot of chatter and noise on social media and over time we follow more and more accounts until it can feel overwhelming. Be picky about who you choose to follow and take time to unfollow and unfriend old accounts that no longer excite you. If you don't want to permanently cut ties with a user, then mute them or unfollow their posts. Make a habit of unfollowing one account every time you follow a new one.

Think about your intention

When you start following someone new, think about what your intention is in doing so. Is it because you want them to see you? Is it because they have something to say that will help you achieve your goals?

LIKE EVERYTHING IN LIFE, SPENDING TOO LONG ON SOCIAL MEDIA CAN BE A PROBLEM. USE IT IN MODERATION – STUDIES HAVE SHOWN THAT IF WE USE IT PROPERLY, TIME SPENT ON SOCIAL MEDIA CAN BOOST FEELINGS OF SELF-ESTEEM

Interact with others

Social media is a great forum for questions and answers. Whether it's joining a Facebook group for like-minded people or using a hashtag to listen in to what people are saying about a certain subject, social media can give you solutions and a new perspective.

Follow accounts that post content that aligns with your goals

If you want to lose weight and get fit, or are starting in a new field of work, for example, follow accounts that offer you valuable advice and help you achieve your goals. It goes without saying that there is a huge amount of brilliant content online, so seek out the information that helps you reach your personal goals and aims.

Connect with mentors

There are many people at the top of their fields on platforms like Twitter and LinkedIn. Seek the people out who you admire, interact with them and if it's appropriate, ask specific questions. Chances are they will be happy to offer you some advice and help!

Read and absorb

Rather than mindlessly scrolling through social media, try to engage and read posts carefully. This should be made easier if you have a social feed full of upbeat and exciting content from minimal accounts.

6.00

7.00

8.00

9.00

10.00

11.00

12.00

13.00

14.00

15.00

16.00

17.00

18.00

19.00

20.00

21.00

22.00

23.00

◄ **10.30 P.M.**

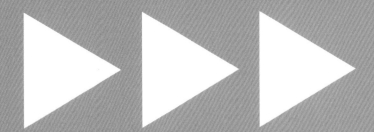

HABIT 7
SLEEP

How often do you take some quiet time out before you go to sleep? Getting enough sleep is the cornerstone of good health, yet recent figures show that we are getting less sleep than ever. Seventy-five years ago, less than 8 per cent of the population were trying to get by on six hours or less sleep per night; now one in two of us is. It's not just the quantity of sleep; it's the quality of sleep that matters. Our busy lives, technology usage and work and family responsibilities are intruding on sleep time and causing a multitude of problems, which undermine the duration and quality of our sleep. This becomes a vicious cycle, where our inability to drift off and sleep properly then becomes the problem. A common myth is that we can 'get by' on not much sleep with no negative effects. Sleep can feel like an indulgence when we are busy and stressed but it's not a luxury; sleep is a necessity.

Ease the transition from wake time to sleep time with a period of relaxing activities around an hour before bed. This theory is often applied to small children and a consistent routine can help you get to sleep quickly too. What works for me might be different for you; I like to do some light reading or maybe a Sudoku. Other ideas include taking a bath – the cooling down of your body afterwards helps you to relax – listening to classical music, meditating or reading.

Scientifically, there are various ways of assessing inadequate sleep and the amount of sleep each individual needs is unique and will depend on a number of factors, including lifestyle, age and health. Most of us should be getting eight to nine hours, while teenagers need more like nine or even ten hours.

Lack of sleep can have profound effects. Perhaps the most visible effect is weight gain because lack of sleep disrupts the two main hormones that control hunger – ghrelin and leptin – leading us to feel hungrier and consume more calories. Sleep also affects how our bodies react to insulin, the hormone that controls our blood glucose levels. This can make us more prone to conditions like type 2 diabetes and heart disease.

Not sleeping enough can also make us vulnerable to infections. A recent study of identical twins at the University of Washington showed that when one twin was sleep-deprived it suppressed their immune system. While the brain sleeps, it also rids itself of harmful toxins that build up during waking hours. This 'waste-removal system' is thought to be one of the main reasons why we sleep and research suggests that chronic poor sleep and failing to clear away toxic proteins increases the risk of brain disorders, such as Alzheimer's or Parkinson's disease.

In addition to this, sleep supports healthy growth and development, consolidates and improves memory, sharpens our attention spans and focus, spurs creativity and improves performance at school and work. It reduces our stress levels and improves our mood. One recent survey of over 8,000 people by the Oxford Economics and National Centre for Social Research found that a healthy amount of sleep was the strongest indicator of living well – and ranked much more highly than a pay rise.

As a child and teenager, when I was away from home I used to sometimes struggle to get to sleep and then for a while, I found it hard before big competitions. But I have a strict sleep routine. I always go to bed and get up at the same time every day, even on the weekends. I make sure my bedroom feels calm and cool and is clear of clutter. All of these ideas are said to feed into good sleep.

I find it useful to note down anything important that I need to do or remember for the next day the night before – even just getting my clothes together or packing ready for a trip means that I won't lie awake worrying that I will forget something! Once you have written these things down, you can completely switch off from your work. Dimming the lights will also send a signal to your body that it is time to relax and fall asleep, so light candles or lower the lights.

IF YOU DO ONE THING ...
Make bedtime a self-care ritual that you look forward to and take time over, with a regular routine that starts at least an hour before your intended bedtime.

7 steps to clean sleep

Hot on the heels of clean eating is the wellness trend 'clean sleeping', a term coined by Gwyneth Paltrow, who said we need to be thinking about our sleep before we tackle our diets. The basic principle of clean sleeping is trying to get seven to eight hours of full sleep a night, free from distractions. Here are some clean-sleeping ideas you could try to incorporate into your routine.

1

Always eat breakfast before you leave home. Experts say the stress of the commute on an empty stomach could affect your sleep that night.

2

Make your bedroom a sanctuary to create a clear association between the space and sleep.

3

Stop looking at your phone at least an hour before you go to bed and ban it from the bedroom!

4

Aim to be asleep at 10.30 p.m. The hours before midnight are said to be the most powerful so make a point of going to bed around this time so your body can access the 90-minute sleep cycle before midnight.

5

Maintain a consistent sleep schedule. This keeps our internal circadian rhythm happy and makes falling asleep easier. Set yourself a sleep schedule; it's fine if you can't go to sleep at the time you set yourself but make sure you get up at the time you originally intended. You will soon find that you will be able to drop off more easily.

6

Give yourself a head or foot massage to relieve tension before bedtime.

7

Minimise stimulants like caffeine and refined sugar throughout the day and avoid caffeinated drinks after 2 p.m.

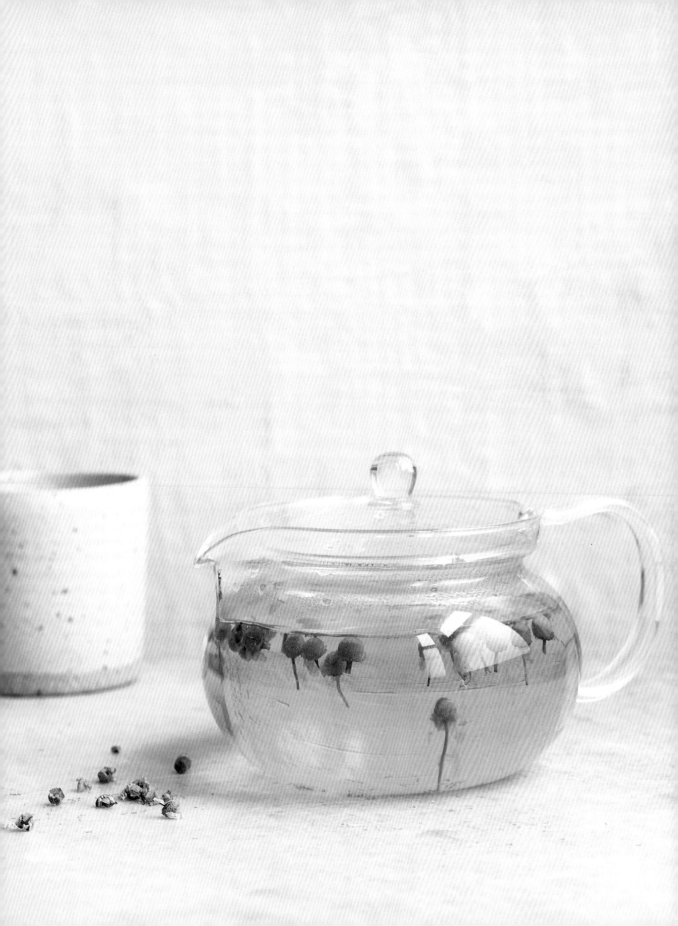

9 Body Scan meditation steps

I always use this exercise to help me fall asleep at bedtime and sometimes I haven't even got past my tummy and I'm asleep! This practice will release tension, quieten the mind and help you develop greater sensitivity and connection with your body. By becoming more attuned to what's happening in your body, you then become better equipped to respond in the right way. Experts say that by doing this exercise regularly, we also can work through pain and difficult emotions more easily. If you find it hard, start by focusing on steps 1–4 in real detail. Once you have practised this, add in the remaining steps.

1

Lie back and take a few moments to check in with your body. Notice the sensations, like the feelings of touch or pressure, sensing the contact your body is making with the mattress.

2

Bring your attention to the natural flow of your breathing. Notice how your abdomen gently rises as you inhale and falls as you exhale. On each out-breath, let your body sink deeper into the bed.

3

Start by focusing on the crown of your head. How does it feel? Are there any sensations like tingling, numbness or tightness? Just become aware, do not try to change any feelings. If you want, imagine tensing and relaxing the areas as you scan, or you can physically tense and relax them – whatever you feel most comfortable with.

4

Bring your attention to the eyes, nose, cheeks, mouth, jaw, tongue, chin, neck and ears. Think about the sounds coming into your ears or the warmth of your mouth.

5

Move your awareness into the neck and shoulders, noticing any tensions in these muscles and releasing these. Feel the parts of your body in contact with the mattress and stretch your awareness into the arms, elbows, wrists, hands and fingers.

6

Now shift your focus to the front of the body – to the chest area, noticing the subtle rise and fall of the chest and thinking about your ribcage and beating heart.

7

Turn your awareness to the abdomen and stomach, then to the back of your body, scanning from your shoulder blades to the middle of your back and then your lower back. Consciously release any tension before moving your awareness to the pelvis, focusing on the hip bones, sitting bones and groin.

8

Now move your attention into the thighs of both legs, down to the knees and into the calves. Finally move your attention into both feet, the arches, the heels, the balls and the tops of the feet.

9

Allow yourself to feel completely relaxed. Continue scanning up and down your body until you drop off!

Simple ways to detox your bedroom space

We spend a third of our lives sleeping and the bedroom is the space that we rest in, so it makes sense to have one that is peaceful, so our bodies and minds can rest and rejuvenate.

Get rid of the devices
Nothing will distract you from sleep as much as a television, iPad or mobile phone. These disrupt our natural sleep cycles because they radiate blue light.

Upgrade your mattress
Look for a mattress and bedding that is made from natural fibres. This is not an area where you should try to save money – buy the best quality you can afford and do your research before making this important purchase. One simple way to make your mattress more comfortable is to get a mattress topper. I find the ideal combination for me is a slightly harder mattress with a mattress topper to soften it!

Reduce the clutter
Your bedroom is the last thing you see at night and the first thing you see in the morning, so by clearing away any mess and clutter, you will improve your mental clarity and well-being – and be able to find things more quickly!

Keep your cool
Most of us think that getting warm and cosy is the key to a good night's sleep but actually the opposite is true. Our bodies cool down naturally at night, increasing the chances of rejuvenating sleep. Keep your bedroom cool and don't shy away from opening a window to let some fresh air in!

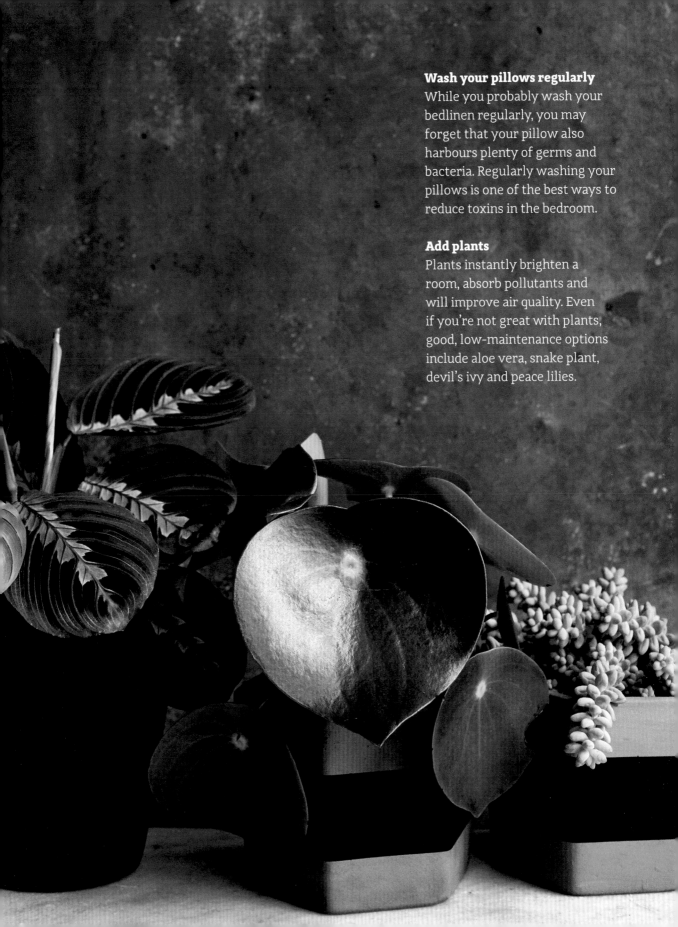

Wash your pillows regularly
While you probably wash your bedlinen regularly, you may forget that your pillow also harbours plenty of germs and bacteria. Regularly washing your pillows is one of the best ways to reduce toxins in the bedroom.

Add plants
Plants instantly brighten a room, absorb pollutants and will improve air quality. Even if you're not great with plants, good, low-maintenance options include aloe vera, snake plant, devil's ivy and peace lilies.

INDEX

ACKNOWLEDGEMENTS

It's amazing to think quite how many people have contributed to the making of this book – it's been a great team effort and I am hugely thankful. Massive thanks to following people:

The team at HQ. To Rachel Kenny, Lisa Milton and Sarah Hammond for their vision; Lily Capewell, Jo Rose and Bengolo Bessala for their PR and marketing prowess.

Emma Marsden and Fiona Hunter for all their assistance with the recipes and nutrition. A big thank you also to Georgina Rodgers for her help and creativity – you are an absolute gem!

To everyone who helped design my book and make it look so fantastic. Louise Leffler, Louise McGrory, Ellis Parrinder, Lou Kenney, Louie Waller, James Yardley and Victoria Penrose. To Adidas, Topman and Diesel for the clothes for this photoshoot.

To the team at James Grant. To my literary agent Rory Scarfe for guiding me with all things book-related, and to Tim Edwards, Holly Bott, Alex McGuire and Mary Bekhait for helping and supporting me every step of the way.

To my diving team. Jane, Grace and Robyn, thanks for putting up with my constant chat about food.

To my family and friends. Sophie, Liam, Joe, Leah, Tom and Simon – thanks for letting me test out some recipes on you at our Monday Night Dinner Club.

To Lance for supporting me through everything and giving me inspiration every day!

HQ
An imprint of HarperCollinsPublishers Ltd
1 London Bridge Street
London SE1 9GF

10 9 8 7 6 5 4 3 2 1

First published in Great Britain by HQ
An imprint of HarperCollinsPublishers Ltd 2018

Text Copyright © Tom Daley 2018

Photography Copyright © Ellis Parrinder 2018

Tom Daley asserts the moral right to be identified as the author of this work. A catalogue record for this book is available from the British Library.

ISBN 978-0-00-828137-3

Our policy is to use papers that are natural, renewable and recyclable products and made from wood grown in sustainable forests. The logging and manufacturing processes conform to the legal environmental regulations of the country of origin. For more information visit: www.harpercollins.co.uk/green

Photography: Ellis Parrinder
Food styling: Lou Kenney
Prop styling: Louie Waller
Clothes stylist: James Yardley
Make-up: Victoria Penrose, Sam Golley
Design: Louise Leffler
Nutritionist: Fiona Hunter, BSc (Hons) Nutrition, Dip Dietetics
Editorial Director: Rachel Kenny
Project Editor: Sarah Hammond
Creative Director: Louise McGrory

Printed and bound in Italy by Rotolito

All rights reserved. No part of this publication may be reproduced, stored in a retrieval system, or transmitted, in any form or by any means, electronic, mechanical, photocopying, recording or otherwise, without the prior permission of the publishers.

This book is sold subject to the condition that it shall not, by way of trade or otherwise, be lent, re-sold, hired out or otherwise circulated without the publisher's prior consent in any form of binding or cover other than that in which it is published and without a similar condition including this condition being imposed on the subsequent purchaser.

The information in this book will be helpful to most people but is not a substitute for advice from a medical practitioner and is not tailored to individual requirements. You should always check with your doctor before starting an exercise programme, particularly if you have not exercised before. The author and publishers do not accept any responsibility for any injury or adverse effects that may arise from the use or misuse of the information in this book.